W9-AMU-799

A Time of Grace

*One Family's Experience
with Chronic Care*

by

Daniel Donovan

Paulist Press
New York *Mahwah*

1990

Copyright © 1990 by Daniel Donovan

All rights reserved. No part of this book may be reproduced or transmitted in any form or by any means, electronic or mechanical, including photocopying, recording or by any information storage and retrieval system without permission in writing from the Publisher.

Library of Congress Cataloging in Publication Data

Donovan, Daniel, 1937–
    A time of grace: one family's experience with chronic care/by Daniel Donovan.
        p. cm.
    ISBN 0-8091-3164-1
    1. Cerebrovascular disease—Patients—Long term care. 2. Aged—Long term care. I. Title.
RC388.5.D636   1990
362.1'6'092—dc20   90-7185
                                                     CIP

Published by Paulist Press
997 Macarthur Boulevard
Mahwah, NJ 07430

Printed and bound in the
United States of America

Contents

In memory of my parents,
Dorothy and Daniel Donovan

1. By Way of Introduction

It was late on a Monday afternoon in March of 1988 that my sister-in-law telephoned with the news that my mother had suffered a stroke and was on her way by ambulance to a local hospital. My initial reaction was one of shock and disbelief. In spite of her eighty-four years it had seemed to me that she still possessed enormous vitality and energy. An independent woman who had lived on her own since my father's death some twenty years earlier, she had continued to play the organ every day at the noon mass in her parish church.

My sense of shock was heightened when I saw her stretched out under a sheet in one of those anonymous and barren cubicles that are the hallmark of emergency wards in large city hospitals. Although intermittently conscious, she was extremely confused. The stroke had been a massive one and had resulted in severe paralysis of the entire left side. As vulnerable and stricken as she appeared I kept thinking of her former strength. Then and later an image came to mind, the image of a felled tree—a majestic creature brought low.

She had suffered the stroke on the previous evening and had lain on the floor of the bathroom of her apartment for close to sixteen hours. Her absence from the noon mass the next day had made people realize that something was wrong. A neighbor who often went with her to church had the caretaker of the apartment building investigate. It was they who found her and raised the alarm.

It was Monday of Holy Week, a day that marks the beginning of that period of the year during which in a special way Christians remember and celebrate the suffering, death,

1

and resurrection of Jesus. My mother's sensitivity to the liturgical year gave the timing of her stroke a certain poignancy. It was something to which she herself would refer.

For days, even for weeks, she continued to hover at the edge of death. There were moments when it seemed inevitable that she would slip over, but somehow she never did. Members of the family took turns in being with her. It was her death about which we thought and with which in our different ways we attempted to come to terms.

Long before she was out of danger, the hospital began the process of looking for a place for her in a chronic care facility. As understandable as this haste was from the point of view of an acute care institution, it left me rather breathless. I knew practically nothing about chronic care, and because I was so concerned about my mother's possible death, I was not able to give much thought to it at the time. I came later to recognize that this had been a serious mistake on my part. Had I gone to the various institutions that were being considered and found out for myself what the options were, the following six months would have been a great deal easier.

Although mother was extremely withdrawn and probably in a state of both shock and depression, she was quite adamant about where she did and did not want to go. Within little more than two weeks she was offered a private room in a local Catholic institution. A combination home for the aged and hospital, my mother knew it well and had at one time even been a member of its board. For some reason that was not clear to me, she refused to go there. She much preferred another facility in spite of the fact that its chronic care units had no private rooms. Located just down the street from where she had lived, she thought that it would be more easily accessible to her friends. She had, moreover, been the president and a long-time member of its auxiliary. Later I thought that she probably underestimated the seriousness of her condition and was hoping that she would be part of its rehabilitation program rather than on one of its chronic care floors. Whatever the reason for her choice, I felt obliged to respect it. When a semi-private room became available there, we moved her to it.

If it was difficult to see my mother at the point of death, it was even more difficult to face the possibility that she might survive for an extended period of time at a drastically reduced level. The emotions I felt on my first visit to the chronic care hospital were overwhelming and unforgettable. The sight of so many elderly and incapacitated people, as sad and depressing as it was in itself, became infinitely more so because my mother was among them. The inscription that Dante had placed over the gate of hell seemed apt: "Abandon hope, all you who enter here."

And yet I did not. There was no time to indulge in personal feelings and reactions. Mother was in greater need than she ever had been before, and it was obvious that if I and others did not do something for her, her last weeks and months would represent a tragic ending to what had been a rich and full and generous life. To suggest some of the ways we tried to help her and how she responded to our efforts will be a central theme of the following pages. At this point all I want is to give an initial sense of the course of her illness and of our involvement in it.

The most positive and encouraging thing that happened over the next few months was what the occupational therapists and physiotherapists were able to do. Although initially it seemed as if mother had been condemned to little more than a vegetable existence, by July she was able to sit up for a few hours each day in a wheelchair, partially feed herself, and respond to some degree to visitors. That she succeeded in coming back as far as she did was a tribute to her determination and residual vitality. She could not, how-

ever, have done it on her own. Family and therapists reinforced one another in supporting and prodding her. We
refused to let her give up.

It was not easy for mother to adjust to chronic care.
What probably made it more difficult for her was the fact
that I and other members of the family felt frustrated in our
efforts to deal with the hospital and with some of its staff. In
spite of the cooperation and kindness of the therapists, we
felt like outsiders. I was often angry at what I took to be
callousness and insensitivity. I remember more than once
coming upon mother in the corridor, in direct view of the
nurses' station, half out of her chair with her table top on
the floor. Although such things can happen easily, they became for me symptomatic of a certain attitude. What out-
raged me most was that there seemed to be no one to whom
we could turn for redress.

During the summer I broached with my mother the
possibility of transferring her to another institution. I asked
her in particular what it was that she had against the Catholic hospital that had originally offered her the private room.
She said that over the years a number of friends of hers had
been there and that they had not liked it at all. If it was bad,
she added, where she was now was even worse. She asked if
she could be moved.

For July and most of August she was fortunate enough
to enjoy a certain privacy. The woman with whom she had
been sharing the room had been transferred to another institution in late June. The new situation made conversation
and listening to music a great deal easier. We were able to
create a special kind of feeling in the room, one that isolated
her to some degree from the depressing atmosphere of the
corridor. Although this clearly helped her, I knew that it was
artificial and brittle. My hope was to move her before someone else arrived. Unfortunately this turned out to be impos-

sible. I was with her near the end of August when an old woman of more than a hundred was wheeled into the room. I felt as if we were being overwhelmed by everything that I had been trying to keep at bay. The next two days were bedlam. The women's two elderly daughters were deaf and tended to shout when they spoke. They insisted that because of their mother's eyes the curtains over the windows had to be closed. In the face of the noise, the confusion, and the darkness, mother visibly began to withdraw. On the third day she suffered a seizure that set her back months.

Once this had happened I redoubled my efforts to have her moved as soon as possible. It was as important for me as for her that it be done and that it be done quickly. I wanted a private room for her, but I also wanted a religious environment. Religion had always meant a great deal to my mother. More than most people, she had lived out her life within the ritual and ethos of Catholicism. It made sense that she should be given the opportunity to end her life in the same kind of environment. Most of all I wanted her in an institution where I would be able to deal in some kind of effective way with the administration. Within two weeks she was offered a private room in that very hospital to which initially she had refused to go. I felt enormously relieved.

From September to Christmas mother was in a state of slow decline. Often confused and totally unable to entertain herself, she seemed to be surviving more than living. At the beginning of January her condition leveled out, and from then until early April her life was qualitatively of a different order. More focused than she had been, she talked with a new openness about herself and her feelings; she enjoyed the small things that we were able to do together. She seemed to have won back a certain, although minimal, joy in life.

I was with her on April 5 when she suffered what medical professionals call a cardiovascular accident. It provoked a rapid deterioration that within thirty-six hours led to her death. She knew that she was dying and she approached it in peace and in trust. The final day and a half gave the family time to realize what was happening and to bid her a final farewell.

A little more than a year had elapsed since the initial stroke. It was an extremely difficult time both for my mother and for me, and yet in spite of everything it was also a time of grace. To my surprise and hers I became actively involved with her in her illness to the point of spending close to two hours every day at the hospital. I came to know and appreciate her in a way that I never had before. It was a deeply human and profoundly moving experience.

My experience, however, was more than personal. Over the time that it lasted I dealt with institutions and with health care professionals as well as with my mother. I saw many things that made me reflect on the place of the elderly and of the chronically ill in our society. Experts tell us that we are an aging population. Chronic care will be a part of the life of an increasing number of us. It is important that we begin now to think about it and about what we can do to make it less threatening and less negative.

The most basic conviction to which I have come has to do with the role of the family. Our public institutions vary. Some are more effective and above all more humane than others. Some tend to view families as intruders while others welcome them. Whatever the case, family involvement is essential. For the chronically ill it can make the difference between mere survival and an existence that is worthy of human beings.

Many of the elderly are abandoned people. In some cases they have no surviving relatives, or, if they do, they live at a great distance. In other instances their families are simply too selfish to care. Often, however, the problem lies elsewhere. People are afraid of hospitals and especially of chronic care facilities. They are afraid of their own vulnerability and mortality. They find it difficult to see parents or friends laid low. Such emotions are all the more crippling because when such people do visit they tend to feel inadequate and frustrated. Not knowing what to do or how to be of help, they go away more angry and depressed than they were before. Such feelings make it more difficult to come the next time. Before long they hardly come at all.

The last year of my mother's life presented an enormous challenge, not only to her, but also to her family. I believe that to a large degree we met that challenge. Because we did, her final months were far more than an unfortunate appendage to the rest of her life. In some sense they brought it to a fulfillment. Looking back now one can say that she lived life in all its phases and that she lived it well. As her parents were there to help her in her childhood, so her family was able to assist her at the end.

I write about her illness and about everything that surrounded it in the hope that what I have to say will be of help to others. I would like in particular to be able to reach those who are in a situation similar to the one I was in. I want to encourage them to become involved with their aging and ill parents in as positive a way as they can. We can make a difference for them and, if we do, we as well as they will be the beneficiaries. I hope that people in general will be stimulated to think about the issues that chronic care raises. Our response or lack of response to the chronically ill reveals a great deal about the kind of society that we are becoming.

As a Catholic and as a priest I have come to a deepened conviction about the importance of the church's ministry to the sick and the elderly. Religious institutions that try to serve such people deserve our support. Those who have lived out their life within the context of the Christian community have every right, if possible, to be supported in their last months and years by institutions that embody the same values and vision. Such institutions, moreover, provide Christian communities with an outlet for concrete and visible witness to the gospel. If activists are looking for the marginalized and the defenseless within western society, one of the best places for them to begin is in our chronic care facilities.

Catholic Christianity has always put a premium on the community dimension of religion. It is one of the reasons why it has insisted so much on common worship. If community experience is to have any meaning, however, it must not cease when members move away from the parish into an institution. It is then more than ever that they need the affirmation and sense of belonging that lived community alone can give.

The following pages will interweave story and reflection on it. Both are essential. I do not write as a medical professional or as a trained psychologist or sociologist. My perspective is that of a son, but of a son who happens to be a priest and a theologian. Inevitably my education and experience lead me to see and interpret events in a somewhat distinctive way. I hope that this will not make what I have to say any less valid or helpful for those with a different background. Aging and death, sickness and caring, family relationships in all their complexity are the stuff of every human life. As particular as my experience was, it is or will be in one way or another the experience of almost everyone.

Life today at every stage brings us into contact with institutions. This tends to become more the case as we grow older and as our health gives way. For some the very word "institution" has negative connotations. It should not. Institutions can, of course, fail to achieve the goals and purposes for which they were created. They can be undermined and distorted in innumerable ways. They remain, for all that, necessary and they have in many cases a potential for great good. It is not always simple, however, to deal with them. The drama of the individual and the institution is played out every day in our culture, in education and in welfare and in large industrial concerns. It is perhaps nowhere more acutely experienced than in the health care system. The individual here is primarily the patient, but it is also the family member who tries to intervene on his or her behalf.

An important part of my involvement with my mother was the variety of relationships that developed between myself as an individual and the different institutions with which I had to deal. I hope that the account of my experiences will provoke those who run our health care facilities to think about the issues that are implied in such relationships. I hope, too, that it will encourage individuals not to be overwhelmed by the difficulties that they might initially encounter. There are ways of dealing with every institution; sometimes it simply takes a little more ingenuity and tenacity before one learns how to do it.

I want to conclude this introduction with a simple word of thanks. It is addressed first of all to the doctors, nurses, and other staff of the three hospitals to which for varying periods of time my mother was confined. In most cases they were both helpful to her and supportive of me and of the rest of the family in our efforts on her behalf. I am particularly grateful to Jane Goodfellow and Mona Rush, a social worker and chaplain respectively, who, by discussing the relevant issues with me and by going over what I wrote, were of real assistance as I tried to clarify my experience and to put it into readable form. The present text is much improved because of their input.

2. Learning To Cope

As much as aging, sickness, and death are a part of life, they are not things about which most of us ordinarily think. This is probably more true of our culture than of many others. In the west in general, and certainly in North America, the elderly and the ill tend to be shunted off into institutions, while death is treated as an arbitrary and intrusive event. It is almost as if we considered such things as an affront to our sense of dignity, an unwarranted imposition on our way of life.

Although I had occasionally thought about the possibility of my mother one day being institutionalized, when it actually happened I discovered that I was not prepared for it at all. Not only did I have to adjust emotionally, but I had to learn a whole set of practical skills in order to be of any real help to her. The most difficult thing initially, however, was learning to cope with the institutions to which she was now confined.

If my mother's illness represented a challenge to me, it was a far greater challenge for her. From one day to the next she lost all ability to look after herself. After being independent for so long, she was suddenly dependent on others for everything. This was as trying for her as facing death or as learning how to live with paralysis. To appreciate her struggle, one has to know something, at least, about her personality and history.

More than anything my mother was an energetic and active person. She was in no sense the stereotypical home-oriented and passive female of her day. As a young woman in the 1920s she left a small Ontario town to come to

10

Toronto on her own. Her first job as a director of a children's choir in St. Paul's parish soon expanded to include what today would be called social work. Before long, financial problems brought her whole family to the city and with them new responsibilities for her. She had to find housing for them and money to help support them.

As serious for her as life was, she always had many friends and knew how to enjoy herself. When I played a tape of "Show Boat" for her in the hospital, she recounted how in the late twenties she had taken a car load of young people to a suburb of Toronto to see it. She could still describe parts of it in detail, including the costumes that the actors wore. Old friends of hers told me how at parties she was always at the piano and how everyone gathered around her to sing.

In the early 1930s she married an Irish Catholic policeman and in what must have seemed a very short time gave birth to three sons. As demanding as the family situation inevitably was, she always found time for other activities. As far back as I can remember she was involved in organizations like the Christian Mothers and the Catholic Women's League. At this, as at every stage of her life, music played an important role. When we were children there always seemed to be young people coming for piano lessons or singers to practice.

As her children became more independent her activity both in the church and in the broader community increased. She worked with the United Appeal, the Red Cross, the Cancer Society, and a host of other charitable associations. Perhaps her most sustained and varied social involvement was with immigration. It began with the Hungarians who came in such large numbers after the failure of their revolution in 1956 and continued with groups from the Caribbean, the Philippines and other parts of the world.

My mother's energy and leadership qualities drew her into positions of responsibility in many of the organizations in which she worked. This in turn brought recognition from both the secular and the church communities. She was especially touched by the Human Relations Award of the Canadian Council of Christians and Jews. Just the third woman to receive that particular award, she accepted it less in her own name than in the name of volunteers in general. She saw herself as part of a wider phenomenon of generous and active people who at the time provided many of the social services that today we regard as part of the government's responsibility.

Like everyone else my mother had her share of grief and pain. When her third son was born, for example, she suffered a severe case of phlebitis and was confined to bed. A doctor at the time predicted that she would never walk again. "Never" turned out to be an exaggeration. A little more than a year later she could be seen making her way up the street to church with the help of a cane.

One of my mother's more striking characteristics was her strength of will. At that time it was probably the most important single factor in getting her back on her feet. In retrospect, it seems clear that it was will power more than anything else that allowed her, in spite of obstacles, to accomplish as much as she did and to keep on going for so long. Will, however, as she eventually learned, has its limits. By itself it cannot cope with death and disability and suffering.

In spite of the popular image of the police, my father was a gentle and kind man, one who was genuinely supportive of his wife and her activities. In his later years he looked after many of the household chores so that she might be free to do things outside of the home. When he died in 1967 my mother lost a real friend and companion as well as a major source of support and encouragement.

What hurt even more than his death was the death from cancer a few years later of her eldest son. Only a mother, I suppose, can appreciate all that it meant to her. Because like so many others of her generation she lacked any real facility in expressing deep personal feelings, it was not easy for her to be with him or to nurse him at the end.

With the approach of her eightieth birthday problems with her legs, perhaps related to the earlier phlebitis, made walking excruciatingly difficult and, for a time, impossible. Here, her will once again made a difference. She refused to give up. As soon as she was able she insisted on getting out, although from then on she had to use a cane and move more slowly than before. It was at this time that she withdrew from most of her activities with the exception of the organ. Almost every day, no matter how she felt, she somehow got herself to the church to play and sing at the noonday mass. For many people in the parish she was "the organist," the embodiment of parish loyalty and dedication.

Through all her life mother had learned to cope. Whatever the challenge, whatever the opportunity, she always found a way to rise to it. Not long before he died my father confided to me his concern about how she would manage financially if she were to survive him. He need not have worried. She coped with that as with everything else—directly, systematically, and successfully.

My mother was always realistic about old age and death. Her will was in order and kept up to date; the funeral arrangements were made and paid for; my power of attorney was renewed as required. Everything that could be done ahead of time to make it easier for us was done. What she could not plan or control was the nature and duration of her final illness. Here, like everyone else, she had to leave it to what for her was not fate or chance but the mystery of divine providence.

Learning to cope with a massive stroke, with chronic care, and with death was the greatest set of challenges that mother ever had to face. There were of course periods of depression and fear, and of longing for release, but they were relatively brief. What most impressed me was the fact that she never seemed to be bitter or angry. When others in the hospital would moan and cry out, she said more than once how much she understood them and that she felt like doing it herself—but she never did.

She obviously did not like being in chronic care any more than other people. She came to accept it, however, with a certain stoicism but also with a touch of grace. The longer she was institutionalized the more she became interested in other patients. She encouraged me to share cookies and candies with those who sat in the corridor near her room. She often asked whether this or that person had gotten her lunch. No matter how badly she felt, she was always able to respond to those who spoke to her and to ask how they were feeling. Her sense that everyone was to be treated with friendliness and politeness was so deeply ingrained as to be a kind of natural reflex.

If learning to cope with what had happened was a challenge for my mother, it was also a challenge for those of us who wanted to be with her and support her. We had to develop ways of relating to and helping her in her weakened and changing state. We also had to learn to deal with the health care system that now stood between her and us. Because of the emotional and other demands that the situation put on us, we had to cope in a new way with ourselves and with one another; in particular we had to be honest about and face our own long-standing relationships with her. Our success or failure in doing all of this would have repercussions not only for ourselves but also for her. Her ability to handle her new situation would depend to a very great degree on what we could do for her. An account, therefore, of how she coped is inseparable from the story of what I and others were able to do.

It is one thing to deal with parents in their own home, it is quite another to relate to them in an institutional setting. Already complex relationships can become even more complicated because they now involve other people, people who both have their own distinctive personalities and who fill institutional roles. The degree, moreover, to which such people allow families to approach them as persons rather than simply as representatives of a bureaucratic structure varies dramatically.

I have nothing but admiration and gratitude for the care that my mother received at the hospital to which she had been taken immediately after the stroke. The doctors and nurses with whom we dealt were both competent and humane. The situation was a critical one, and they were understanding and supportive. The experience in the emergency ward, however, had been somewhat less encouraging. The staff was obviously very busy but also somewhat defensive. A simple effort to elicit information was rebuffed in a way that made me feel like someone who had no right to be there.

Most of us approach health care institutions with a certain trepidation. They represent a world that is other than the world of everyday experience; it is a world that has its own rules and regulations, its own rituals and ethos. Because it deals with sickness and health, life and death, it has an emotional quality about it that is unique. This makes it doubly intimidating. The people who work there are the anointed ones, and we who come to them for service are the laity. They are in a position of power, and we of weakness. Every advantage is on their side. Although they do not always seem to appreciate it, the onus is on them to take the first step and to reach out to us, whether we be patients or families of patients. If medical people are too busy or if their personalities are such as to make it impossible for them to do so, others must do it for them.

Once my mother was actually admitted to the hospital our relationship to the staff was excellent. They accepted our presence and involvement, and our opinions were sought and treated with respect. The social worker assigned to us was very helpful on a personal level. She had a wonderfully direct way of dealing with people and was the first to draw my mother out explicitly on the prospect of dying. When I expressed my admiration for the way she had done this, she said that it was something that when she first began working in a hospital she would have been incapable of doing. A stint of several years in Nigeria, where death is experienced very much as a part of life, had made it easier for her to be open about it.

I have already said how the seriousness of my mother's condition and the intensity of the emotions it provoked focused my thoughts and concerns and those of the family on her probable death. It hardly seemed possible at the time that she would survive. This was the opinion of doctors and nurses as well as our own. The issue of long term care was upon us before we were ready to deal with it. Within a little more than three weeks of the stroke, mother was on her way to the chronic care facility for which she had expressed a preference.

It was difficult for me to face the fact that my mother was in chronic care. The initial sight of her in that context was devastating. My feelings of vulnerability and inadequacy were heightened by the absence of any outreach to me on the part of the institution and its representatives. Although I was there every day at noon hour, no one in any position of authority approached me during the entire first week. When I finally inquired about a prognosis and a program for her I was told rather curtly that she was an old woman who had suffered a serious stroke.

Whatever the reason for the institution's inadequacy, I now realize that I should have exercised more initiative and sought out the person in charge the first day. That I failed to do so is not surprising given my emotional state at the time. As understandable as it might have been, however, my neglect colored the whole subsequent experience.

After my mother had been there a week, I confronted a doctor who had been called in because of some congestion that she was experiencing. I explained that no one had volunteered any information to me or other family members and that my attempt to discover what might be done for her had provoked the response that it did. This was unacceptable, I said, and although I was realistic about her condition, I wanted some kind of therapy if only for morale reasons. He was surprised to learn that the stroke had only taken place a month earlier. The delay in finding chronic care places often means that when people with strokes do arrive at such institutions it is at such an advanced stage of their illness that staff feel justified in approaching them from an almost exclusively custodial perspective.

It was only later that I realized how anomalous my first experience of chronic care had been. Although the institution possessed a social work department, there were no social workers available for the chronic care units. Nor was there any program offered to families introducing them to the institution and its services. Nothing was done in my case to help me understand my mother's condition; no suggestions were made about what I might do in order to be of some assistance to her. The message that all this gave me was that I and families in general were not looked upon in a favorable light. Probably perceived as possible threats to the routine and good order of the institution, we were tolerated rather than welcomed.

What was true of families seemed also to be true of volunteers. A nun in the parish where my mother had lived wanted to get together a small group of parishioners who would be willing to take turns in helping with meals. Instead of talking directly to me, she unfortunately asked the hospital chaplain to approach the unit administrator who rejected the offer. The reason given was that it would take time to train such people. If family members wanted to help feed my mother, they were acceptable, but others were not. All this meant, in the end, was that I had to find my own volunteers.

The more I thought about all of this, the less sense it made, and that from every point of view, including the economic. Mounting deficits are bringing pressure on governments to cut back in the area of health care. This is already having its effect in chronic care facilities. Even minimal experience in such places reveals the problem of understaffing. Families and volunteers can be of help here. The simple fact, for example, of being with a patient at a meal time relieves a staff member to do something else.

The most important reason, however, for encouraging families to become involved is not economic but therapeutic. Only close friends and relatives know much about the life, accomplishments, and interests of the elderly. Building on that knowledge they can reinforce their sense of identity by recalling and affirming their pasts. The very presence, moreover, of such people communicates to the chronically ill that they are not forgotten or abandoned but that they remain valued and cherished for themselves.

If the elderly and the incapacitated are viewed primarily as physical specimens to be kept clean and to be fed and to be given necessary medical care, their families will inevitably be perceived as outsiders, as possible threats to the professional routine. If patients, however, are cherished as human beings with a fundamental dignity and with basic rights including the right to a human environment and to human contact, then families will be recognized as an integral part of care-giving.

The fact that the institution to which my mother was confined seemed as unwelcoming as it did created in me a profound sense of mistrust. This meant that instead of simply concentrating on her condition and on what I could do to alleviate it, I was constantly worrying about what might happen to her when I was not there. The experience was not unique to me. It was one that family and friends shared. Members of six or seven other families who had a relative in the same institution spoke to me of similar concerns at one time or other during the almost six months that mother was there.

In spite of the difficulty, I had no intention of giving up. I came every day at noon and saw to it that someone else was there for the evening meal. This kind of dedication soon began to have an impact on the staff. By affirming the importance in my eyes of caring for my mother I was affirming the importance of the work that the nurses and therapists themselves were doing. This was appreciated. Nursing assistants, in particular, have a difficult and thankless job, one that is not highly valued even from a monetary point of view. Learning names, greeting people with a smile, occasionally bringing a gift of fruit or candy: such gestures made a difference. Slowly, almost surprisingly, there developed a sense of collaboration, of being part of a team. Without realizing it, I was learning how to cope in what seemed initially to be a rather forbidding environment.

This sense of teamwork marked the relationship with the occupational therapists and physiotherapists almost from the beginning. As overworked as they were, they were delighted to meet a family that was so involved and that was so appreciative of what they were trying to do. It helped considerably that a cousin, herself a medical doctor, was able to come almost every morning throughout the summer. She saw to it that my mother was up and often took her down to therapy herself.

The stroke affected the whole of the left side. In the beginning the paralysis of both arm and leg as well as the general weakness of the body was considerable. With time and exercise she was able to sit up for increasing lengths of time; a certain vitality came back into the leg but never enough for even minimal walking. The left arm and hand remained quite inert as long as she lived. As with so many people with strokes, mother had to relearn many of the simple things that she had learned as a child: how to use a spoon, how to feed herself, how to drink from a cup. In all of this we reinforced and supported the therapists, and they in turn encouraged and helped us. Their enthusiasm was a breath of air in an otherwise stifling and depressing atmosphere.

The decision to move my mother to another institution was partly motivated by the positive things that I hoped we would find there and partly by a desire to escape the situation in which she then was. One of the things we wanted was a private room. For some people in chronic care, especially for those who have few visitors, a shared room, for all its other drawbacks, can at least mean a little less isolation. This was not a major issue with my mother. It was clear by this time that family and friends were committed to visiting on a regular basis. A single room would guarantee some quiet and would permit her to listen to music without disturbing others. More importantly it would provide the atmosphere without which relaxed and spontaneous conversation can scarcely take place.

I also wanted her to be in an environment that would be more open to religious values. As it turned out this became an important factor in helping her cope both with her disability and with death. For myself, I wanted to be able to start again with another institution, one that would be more welcoming to families, one in regard to which I could be a little more trusting.

In order that all of this would have some chance of being realized, I visited the second institution twice before making any application to move my mother there. The first visit was to a resident who had formerly been in the hospital where my mother then was. She was able to give me a good overview of the place from her perspective. The second visit was more formal. A friend put me in touch with the public relations officer who took me on a tour of the building and introduced me to some of the staff. With these two visits I had a sense that this time I had a good idea of the institution with which we were getting involved.

The difficulties that I encountered in having the transfer papers completed and forwarded epitomized the more negative aspects of my relationships to the first facility. I contacted the social work department and asked them to initiate the procedures. They answered that as they had no representative on the floor, I would have to address my request to the head nurse or to the doctor. My letter to the latter was acknowledged a day later. He assured me that the process was already underway.

Twice, at ten day intervals, I went to the social work

department to inquire how the procedure was going and to prod them to hasten it along. Both times I was told that everything was in order and that it was just a matter of time. Ten days after the second visit—a month, in other words, after the original request—a nurse on the floor handed me the application papers. Although filled out a month earlier, they had never left the nurses' station. A final call to the head of social work brought an apology and the recommendation that I bring the papers to be copied and then deliver them myself that afternoon. Although the medical data was now a month out of date, I seized the opportunity and did what had been suggested. In the end it took a matter of hours to accomplish what in the institution's hands had set us back a month.

The move brought new challenges, especially for my mother. If she had been confused before, she was even more confused now. It took her weeks to adjust to the different surroundings, the new routines, the strange faces. Gradually, however, she did, until finally she felt as much at home there as one can feel in such a place.

This was a more open institution in regard to families than the other one had been. It must of course be added that by this time I had accumulated a certain experience and had learned something about dealing with hospital professionals. However much that counted for me, here there was clearly a tradition for involving families and for assisting them to understand and to cope with the problems of the elderly and of those in chronic care. A key role here belonged to the social workers, one of whom was assigned to each floor. Part of their task is to meet with family members, to help them deal with their feelings and concerns, and to suggest ways that they might continue to support their recently admitted relative. They try to elicit information from families about the patient's background and interests, information that could be helpful for the staff in developing a therapeutic program.

The social work department in the facility periodically offers a series of seminars for families. The topics treated include the aging process, typical illnesses with which the elderly are confronted, forms of therapy, and the various programs offered by the institution. Speakers encourage families to remain involved and they suggest ways of coping with some of the problems they will inevitably meet. Given the nature of chronic care institutions the presence of social workers seems essential if a positive relationship between family and professional staff is to be established and maintained. It was their absence on the chronic care floors of the first institution that compounded the difficulty there. In answer to a query I was told that this unfortunate situation was due to fiscal restraint.

The key person in the running of the various units into which the hospital is divided is the unit administrator. A senior nurse, her responsibility embraces all the activity that takes place on her floor. She more than anyone else sets the tone for staff, patients, and families in the unit and is the person to whom one turns for authoritative action. The head of my mother's unit was a direct and forthright woman who made amply clear from the beginning her desire to be available and to respond to problems or concerns that might arise.

As it turned out, learning how to cope with the institutional elements this second time around was not difficult. It was, in fact, almost a matter of common sense. Most things one could do oneself. It was extremely rare that I had to ask the unit head to intervene, and when I did the results were immediate and positive.

Small things inevitably happened. If the relationship with the unit administrator had been a negative one, they might well have developed into serious problems. Two examples can illustrate what I mean. It was important to me that my mother be gotten up every day for a couple of hours around noon. Not only was the change a good thing for her, but it created the possibility for a much better visit. An additional reason for having her up on Sundays was to enable her to be taken to mass. On the first two weekends she was left in bed. When I questioned the nurses as to why this was the case, they told me that her wheelchair had disappeared both times. Once I brought this to the attention of the unit head, it never happened again.

After some trial and error it became evident that the most practical clothing for my mother was the track suit. Although we had a few skirts in her closet, I put a sign up inside of it requesting that she be dressed in a track suit. When people persisted in using the skirts, I put a second sign on the door. The next day I arrived to find her sitting in her wheelchair under the sign dressed in a skirt. When I asked the nurse why she had not put a track suit on her, she said that because my mother had had bowel care that day, the skirt was more convenient.

I went to the unit head and sought her advice. Given the fact that my mother was often cold, what kind of clothing, I asked her, would be suitable. A track suit, she answered. When I then told her my story, she assured me that I would have no further difficulty. She was right.

Both of these examples have to do with what in themselves are small things. Yet it is precisely such things that, depending on the way they are handled, can add up to a positive or negative experience. It was in terms of the confidence and freedom that I felt in addressing such small issues that I came to appreciate the difference between the two hospitals.

Communication is central to any successful relationship between individuals and an institution. It is crucial that the means of communication be there and that everyone know what they are and how they work. More than anything else it is the absence of communication or its breakdown that makes such relationships tense and frustrating.

Because families at the outset are in the emotional state that they are, and because most of them have so little experience with chronic care facilities, the responsibility for establishing lines of communication and for making them known resides with the institution. Once that has been done, the family has its own responsibility. It has to enter into the process and, while respecting the nature of the institution and the work load of its staff, to make known courteously but clearly its concerns and desires. It is only if a genuine respect between staff and family develops that the experience can be a positive one, one that truly serves the needs of the chronically ill.

Hospitals, like so many institutions, are often barren and impersonal. Their architecture and their routine tend to undermine individuality and to reduce people to a common denominator. One of the reasons I wanted a private room for my mother was the hope that by doing something with it, it might become distinctive and to some degree reflective of her personality. To this end I hung on its walls a number of things of both religious and artistic quality along with a collage of family photos. The single most important item of this nature in the room was a picture of her seated at a church organ. It had been taken a few years earlier to mark her fortieth anniversary as organist at Holy Name parish.

The point of the decoration as well as of the plants and flowers that were always in abundance was to create an atmosphere that would reinforce my mother's sense of herself and of her dignity. Everything that was done with the room, however, was also done for the staff and for visitors.

It was crucial that those who had never known her would realize that she was someone who had accomplished a great deal with her life, that as incapacitated as she now was she had been a person of substance.

During the fall, the local Council of Catholic Charities celebrated its seventy-fifth anniversary. To mark the occasion, awards of merit were given to six or seven people who had been active in its work over the years. My mother was one of them. Because the institution in which she now was belonged to the Council and was benefiting from its support, I thought that it would be helpful to add the award to the other things that we already had in her room.

It was important for visitors to be able to cope with mother's condition and with the hospital environment. Some of her old friends never came, and some who did found it hard to deal with her in her reduced state. The atmosphere of the room was meant to facilitate their feeling at home, relaxing, and overcoming their inhibitions. My hope was that they would recognize that in spite of all that had happened it was still the same person who was there and who now needed their friendship and understanding more than ever.

Whenever I came for the evening meal, especially during the winter months when it was already dark by 4:30, I lit a candle in the window. It radiated a feeling of warmth and of life. Its scent was enough to dissipate the kind of odors that are associated with a hospital. To light a candle is a simple gesture, but like so many other small things it helped both mother and me to make the best of a difficult situation.

If I had to learn to cope with my mother's illness and with the institutions to which she was now confined, I also had to juggle a few things in my own life in order to find the time to be with her every day. Unlike many people my responsibilities allow a certain flexibility in my schedule. As a professor at the university the actual number of hours in class are limited. Much time is spent in research and in preparing lectures, in committee work and in consultation. By rearranging everything I created a space in the middle of the day for my visits.

We all have to decide, given our other responsibilities, what we can do. From the beginning, partly because her need was so obvious and partly because it did not seem probable that she would survive all that long, I committed myself to being there daily at one meal and to getting someone else to be there at the other. Because my brother's schedule was much less flexible than mine he was ordinarily only able to come on the weekends. Other relatives and friends graciously filled in on the other days.

It is not pleasant to have to organize other people's generosity, and yet some element of organization is essential. To have several people visit one day and no one else the rest of the week is not very helpful. Every one involved has to commit himself or herself for specific days and times. Although for some that poses a threat to their sense of freedom, if they could bring themselves to do it, they would soon discover that it had become part of their routine.

A nurse once expressed surprise that I was able to be there as often as I was. I asked her what she had done when her children were small. The comparison struck home. She recognized the parallel between what I now was doing and what she had done years before.

The analogy between the situation of children and that of the elderly is not far-fetched. As infants we are totally dependent on others. As we mature we become more independent until the day when we begin the cycle again. We experience in regard to our own children the same responsibility our parents accepted on our behalf. Old age ordinarily brings a progressive loss of independence. This can be heightened dramatically by a serious stroke or by some other comparable illness. The circle is then complete. We now have an opportunity to do for our parents what they once did for us.

The focus of these reflections has been to some extent on the institution and on the need of family members to learn to cope with it. The difficulties and the possibilities in this area are considerable and should be for administrators and planners an object of continuing review. The ability or lack of it on the part of families to deal with the hospital and its representatives can make a real difference in the way that they experience the institutionalization of one of their members. More importantly, what they are able or unable to do can have a substantial impact on the well-being of the chronically ill.

All that I went through with my mother has convinced me of the unique contribution that families are called to make when one of their members enters a chronic care facility. The good they can do is truly enormous. For this reason health care professionals must reach out to them and facilitate their becoming involved. Families, for their part, must respond to the invitation and under no circumstances allow institutional or personal barriers to block or undermine their efforts.

3. Becoming Involved

As daunting as learning to cope with the institutions sometimes was, the real focus of my concern and activity throughout the year was obviously my mother. In the beginning it was in some ways easier to come to terms with her possible death than with her survival. As definitive and difficult as the parting of death is, it is at least clear in its implications. We could, moreover, console ourselves that she had lived a full and productive life. Chronic care, on the other hand, would mean a radically reduced existence for her. It would also, I realized intuitively, touch me in ways that I could not then suspect. The quality of the new stage it opened in her life would depend to a very great degree on the extent to which family and friends would be willing to become involved in it.

I have already said how debilitating for me the initial sight of my mother in chronic care was. The feelings it evoked were above all those of sadness and pity. It was depressing to think that this woman who had been so full of energy and vitality, who had always been so independent, might have to go on living for some indefinite period in such a state. Fortunately, the impulse to reach out and help was sufficiently strong in me that I did not allow such emotions to become crippling. I became involved and by doing so began what to my continuing surprise turned out to be a uniquely enriching and humanizing experience. This was something that at the outset I could never have predicted.

Guilt presents a serious problem for some people when a parent or spouse goes into chronic care. This is particularly true for those who have supported and nursed such a person over a period of gradual decline. It is difficult for them to admit that the day has finally come when they can no longer do what they had done in the past. It is important that people who experience such feelings be helped from the outset to deal with them. Chronic care puts so many demands on us that we cannot afford to have our strength sapped by emotional turmoil of this kind. Social workers can do a real service by helping those who are burdened with such feelings to deal with them.

Guilt was not among the many emotions that I experienced in relation to my mother's situation. The stroke had been so massive and her condition had continued to be so precarious that there was no viable alternative to her being in an institution. As she began to improve she often asked me to take her home, but realistically this was not an option.

Beyond assisting families to overcome unreasonable and paralyzing guilt, people in chronic care facilities need to be creative and persuasive in drawing them into a continuing involvement in the care of their institutionalized member. The chronically ill need their family more than ever. This is something that has to be spelled out and made clear for all concerned. No matter how efficient chronic care hospitals and homes are, no matter how dedicated their staff is, they can only do so much. Far from being shameful to admit such limits, it makes good institutional sense to do so. It is only when people are honest about what can and cannot be done that expectations can be realistic and that compensating activity can be undertaken.

The parallels between chronic care and the educational system are striking. To hand over to professionals all responsibility for the moral, intellectual and social development of children and young people is naive in the extreme. Without effective cooperation between school and family we can be sure that the educational process will not produce the kind of persons that we think it should. The situation with the care of the chronically ill is analogous. Although the contributions of family and institution are different, both are essential. Only when all parties involved fulfill their respective responsibilities will chronic care be able to look after the whole person.

Because families have so much to offer, health care professionals must respectfully and tactfully challenge them to support and be with as much as possible the person being admitted to the institution. The challenge, however, if it is to do any good, needs to be supplemented by specific suggestions that will help the family organize itself and decide what concretely its various members might do.

There is a certain amount of information about the institution and how it works as well as about the general phenomenon of aging and of chronic care that all families need to hear. This information should be communicated in a clear and comprehensible way; ideally its highlights, at least, should be available in written form. This, however, is really only the first step. The chronic care patient is a unique and distinctive person, an individual with ordinarily a whole lifetime of experience and achievement. Any program of activity that is going to help that patient has to emerge from a bringing together of institutional resources and family knowledge. The initiative here normally should be on the side of the chronic care facility.

If families and individuals are going to be able to sustain involvement with the chronically ill over any length of time they will have to discover ways of relating to them that are helpful and that to some degree are capable of becoming a routine. The importance of a relatively fixed pattern of activities only became obvious to me when I had established one. To have to begin all over again each time that one comes is exhausting. Nor is it all that helpful for the person being visited. Like most of us the elderly enjoy and feel reinforced by habit every bit as much as they enjoy the occasional break from it.

What is especially important for visitors of all kinds is that they have a sense that what they do is of value and that it makes a difference. Without such a conviction it is extremely difficult to keep coming back. Sometimes we just have to believe that what we are doing is worthwhile. At other times we know it to be so. Everything, of course, becomes qualitatively easier the moment that we realize that our parent or spouse understands what we are doing and is grateful for it. Such a moment has to be cherished as the special moment of grace that it is.

I had never thought of any of this before my mother's stroke, nor did anyone speak to me about it at the time. What I learned, I learned by doing. Whatever truth there is in what I am writing, it represents my own experience and my reflections on it. I did what I did spontaneously and intuitively. What did not seem to work or feel right I changed or dropped. What I felt at ease with and what my mother seemed to respond to I kept doing. Eventually we had a routine that she looked forward to and that made my being there not a chore but a joy.

While she was still at the acute care hospital, I began what turned out to be a fixed pattern. I usually came at noon in order to help her eat. At that early stage of her illness she was totally incapable of feeding herself. Because the stroke had affected even her ability to swallow she could only eat and drink very slowly. The nursing staff did not have the time that she required, and so it made sense for me to be there.

Her initial reaction to hospital food was decidedly negative. She refused to eat it. As a priest living in an institution I had very little access to any kind of cooking facilities and so I turned to friends who prepared things that would be both nourishing and easy for her to swallow. Then and later my own friends, in many cases people who did not know my mother at all, were wonderfully generous in their support.

Although by the time she was moved to the second chronic care facility she was able to some degree to feed herself, I kept coming at the same time. It continued to make a difference. Not only was I with her but I was able to help her eat at her own slow pace. It was, moreover, a time of day when she was brightest and when therefore talk came most easily.

In a hospital and especially in a chronic care situation, little things can mean a great deal. Although by then accustomed to institutional food my mother enjoyed the fact that there were always homemade cookies and some form of chocolate available if she wanted them. It was an added bonus that she was able to offer them to visitors and staff. It made her feel just a little bit more in command, a little bit more at home.

By being there throughout the meal I could keep the tea warm, encourage her to eat a little more, and bring a touch of cleanliness and dignity to the whole ritual. It was because I could see the difference that my presence made that I persisted in trying to have someone with her at supper every day as well. Here we were extremely fortunate in being helped on a regular basis by a long-time friend of my mother. She insisted again and again that she enjoyed coming and that she got as much from it as she gave.

I have already mentioned how important music was in my mother's life. She played the organ in one parish or another from the time she was fourteen until the day of her stroke. When she was younger she sang in a variety of choirs and accompanied others on the piano. She enjoyed classical music and until she was incapacitated continued to attend symphony concerts and to go to the opera. A neighbor in her apartment building told me how much she missed hearing her in the morning playing Beethoven piano sonatas.

Within days of her stroke and long before any kind of sustained conversation was possible I brought a Walkman and tapes of some of the music that I knew she loved, and played them for her. Because at that time she had a semiprivate room, we used earphones so as not to disturb her roommate. It was difficult to know how much my mother really heard and what effect it had on her, but when I asked if she would like me to put a tape on, she invariably said yes. What at the time she most wanted to hear were classical settings of traditional religious hymns like Schubert's "Ave Maria," Franck's "Panis Angelicus" and Gounod's "O Divine Redeemer." We played these and other favorite pieces repeatedly throughout the year. Their very repetition was like a refrain marking the successive stages of her illness.

After she had been in chronic care for several weeks, she was able to sit up in a wheelchair. Once she had grown accustomed to the chair, I took her one day to the auditorium to see what she could do with one hand on a piano. I was astounded at how well she played. After only a few moments, however, the concentration that was required totally exhausted her.

Relatives lent us an electric keyboard and together we played a number of hymns, with me picking out the simpler melody and she with the right hand filling it out with the appropriate chords. It was not easy for her, but it gave her a certain sense of accomplishment and established connecting links with the past. It also made some of the staff aware for the first time that she had been a musician.

In the early weeks music was very much a part of her dreams and fantasies. She often told me that the choir had been at her apartment the night before and that they had been practicing for Holy Week. Sometimes when I arrived in the morning she asked whether we still had time to get to church so that she could play at the noon mass.

Once she had the private room, we were able to do away with the earphones. Music now became much more important, not only for her but also for me. It was something that we could both enjoy, something that we could share and talk about. It was often while we were doing this that she came to speak about herself and about her past. Her recall of incidents from her childhood and youth astonished me by their clarity and by their content. I remember, for example, her account of one of her first encounters with a certain kind of clericalism. Still a teenager, she was playing the organ in her parish and was accused by the pastor of some kind of mistake in regard to the music. When she defended herself, he simply got angry. This was the beginning for her, she said, of learning how to deal with priests.

Like my mother I, too, love music. In fact I like much of the same music that she did. To be able to listen to it in her hospital room somehow made that room other than it was. Like the art work and the photos on the walls it transformed it into something welcoming and home-like. It made it easier for me to be there.

The Christmas music we listened to included traditional and classical pieces, but in every case it was well played and well sung. The atmosphere it created reached beyond her room. Nurses commented on it, and other patients sometimes stopped their wheelchairs in front of the door in order to listen. It was symbolic of what a family can mean in that kind of institutional setting. Like music, a caring attitude cannot be restricted to a single room. It inevitably touches others.

Early January marked a change in my mother's condition. After a long period of slow decline she leveled off and seemed to have adjusted to her situation. As she did so she became more focused and more capable of sustained conversation. Whether or not it was by chance, the change coincided with a shift in the music to which we were listening. I began bringing tapes of operas that she had known and enjoyed. Because of their dramatic stories and flamboyant characters it was easier for me to talk with her about them than about pure music.

I remember her reaction to Puccini's "La Bohème." That day she seemed more confused than usual. She not only was not sure where she was, she was not even clear whether I was myself or my brother. I put on the tape and asked her if she remembered the opera's opening scene. She proceeded to describe it in detail. After a few minutes she looked up from her food and told me to listen closely because in a moment we would hear one of the most beautiful of all soprano arias. She was, of course, right.

On subsequent days we listened to and talked about "Carmen" and "Aida," "die Walküre" and "Turandot." The conversations were rich and detailed and in many ways deeply revealing. She told me what she liked and what she disliked, and why. The character and action of the proud and harsh Turandot occasioned a remarkable exchange about women and about why it is that if they want to be public persons and accomplish something with their lives they have to have a touch of toughness about themselves. These were things about which it had never before occurred to me that we might one day talk. As is so often the case with parents and children, I came in the end to realize that my mother had had a far richer and more interesting life than I had thought.

Music was a real godsend for my mother in her illness. It related her in a positive way to much that she had experienced and done. By stimulating her memory it reinforced her sense of continuity and identity. As a present aesthetic experience it enabled her to rise at least temporarily above both her surroundings and her situation. On many an occasion it functioned as a deeply personal form of prayer.

One day around Christmas she announced that on the previous evening she had been to a wonderful concert, one that had been put on just for her. She mentioned a man who used to be in one of her choirs and said that he had brought her back to the hospital afterward. I had learned by then that most of her fantasies made some kind of sense even if it was only the sense of dreams. In them I could often discern her hopes and desires as well as her fears and premonitions.

As I was wondering what this particular fantasy was all about, a nurse arrived and told me that the night before a man had visited and had played the violin for her.

Always a reader, my mother became even more of one as she grew older. The more difficult it was to get around and to do other things the more she turned to books. She enjoyed crime stories and historical fiction and some of the nineteenth century masters of the classical novel.

One of the unfortunate results of the stroke was that she could no longer read. Her left eye was all but useless and although she could see with the other one, it was difficult for her to focus, especially on a printed text. When I tried to get her to read something, her right eye tended to stop halfway across the page. The effort became so frustrating for her that I soon gave it up.

Once she was in chronic care I began reading to her, and before very long it became part of our routine. Initially I chose things that I knew that she had already read and that therefore would not be too demanding. We began with Agatha Christie's *Murder on the Orient Express* and continued with her *Death on the Nile.*

She loved to have me read to her. At times I thought she

was asleep, but more often than not she was listening and would suddenly question my pronunciation or make a comment about a character or an incident. The reading stimulated her and gave her something to think and dream about. It also gave us another thing to do together. As with children and with many other people, reading to the chronically ill can have a deep emotional significance. It is not simply a matter of reading a text, and above all not a matter of hurrying through it in order to finish a story. It is, rather, an intense and personal way of being together, of focusing one's attention on one another, of sharing a common activity. Reading has a special meaning for children partly because of the emotional atmosphere that it presupposes and fosters. The same can be true for the elderly and the chronically ill. It provides, moreover, a context for talking about things that really matter but in a way that is not too personal. They enter the conversation as they come up in the story and are talked about in terms of its characters and their situations.

The key in reading to others, whatever their age, is to find things that both reader and listener can enjoy. One day mother made a passing remark about how when she was a child her mother had read her *The Tales of the Arabian Nights*. She answered affirmatively when I asked if she would like to hear them again. As we were reading them it struck me that they were hauntingly suitable. Like the story-telling princess of the tales, my mother, too, needed something to which she could look forward on the next day, something that would keep death at bay.

The last book we read or rather partially read was Tolkien's *The Hobbit*. Although she had heard of it, she had never read it. She laughed at and perhaps even identified with the somewhat bourgeois hobbit with his risky taste for adventure. As we read, it occurred to me that once again the story was an apt one. Like the hobbit, my mother, too, had embarked on a journey, one that had already taken her through the physical and psychological equivalents of dark forests, narrow mountain paths, and cavernous ravines. I wondered how many more trials she would have to endure before coming to the great treasure mountain in the east. *The Hobbit,* like most good children's literature, evokes universal themes.

Whenever possible we did our reading in a large open foyer at the front of the building as far away psychologically from the hospital wing as we could get. In some chronic care institutions it is extremely difficult to escape the hospital atmosphere. This was not the case here, and it was a very positive factor indeed. It was always an incentive for her to finish her lunch so that we could "go for a walk," so that I could wheel her out to the front area.

A small but important element in our walks was the wheelchair. It was a problem almost from the beginning. At every stage of her illness it had to be adjusted. After Christmas when she was no longer able to use it we had to replace it with a lounge chair. As comfortable as this was for her, I found it difficult to handle. A chaplain mentioned a new type of chair, a very flexible and light one, that was reported to be both comfortable and easy to maneuver. Unfortunately there were few such chairs in the institution. After trying and seeing how effective it was, I bought and donated one with the understanding that my mother would be able to use it as long as she lived. She found it comfortable, and I found it very easy to manage.

An extremely helpful side-effect of our walks was contact with a wider variety of people. Almost every day we ran into someone, whether resident or visitor, who knew me or my mother and who stopped for at least a moment to chat. A repeated friendly hello to those we did not know gradually built up among us a neighborly feeling that appealed to my mother's innate gregariousness.

Here, too, little things can make a considerable difference. A bright and distinctive shawl and an attractive blanket seem to announce a desire to be in conversation with others. This, at least, is what happened to us. Over the months innumerable people were able to overcome whatever reticence and shyness they had by remarking on the color or pattern of one or the other. It is almost as if in such an institution people experience themselves in their common humanity in a new way. Even the most modest gesture can win a response.

Our noontime sorties almost always included a stop in the chapel. That there was one in the facility at all was a great boon for my mother. Sacred space had been a large part of her life. After music, architecture has perhaps the greatest spiritual potential of all the arts. From primitive mystic circles marked out by stones to the great Gothic cathedrals of medieval Europe and to the thousands of churches and chapels that dot the North American countryside, space has been shaped, enhanced, and dedicated to what untold generations have cherished as their most sacred acts. The permanence of such structures affirms the permanence of the values that they were built to signify and foster. The church building had always been for my mother a kind of second home.

Blessing ourselves with holy water as we entered the chapel, we invariably went up to the first pew. She liked to see the altar and the decorations that signalled the changing seasons of the liturgical year. Although she sometimes confused where we were with other churches in which she had been in the past, she knew it for what it was and was consoled and affirmed by being there.

Part of our ritual was to pray together. Usually we

would say an Our Father, a Hail Mary, and a Glory Be to the Father. In Lent she liked to make the stations of the cross. I pushed her slowly around the chapel as she recalled and announced the title of each of our fourteen stops. The first time we did it was enormously touching. I was struck by her reserve and awe for the person of Christ. She never used the name "Jesus" but always referred to him simply as "he." Her emotions came out in her references to Mary, when, for example, she said: "He meets his holy and sorrowful mother," and "Taken down from the cross, he is placed into the hands of his compassionate mother." Both of these statements were accompanied by a sob and a shudder. The more often we did the stations, the more contained her emotions became. The practice, however, was clearly a healing and soothing one for her. For me, it was extremely moving.

These were the things that over the months slowly developed into a more or less fixed pattern. I ordinarily arrived just as the lunch was being distributed. Because I was so regular she persisted in believing for the longest time that somehow I was responsible for providing the food for the whole unit. As I set it up and helped her eat, we listened to music and talked about it and about whatever else came to mind. As soon as she was finished we set out on our walk, she regularly reminding me not to forget "our book." If there was sun we would try to find a place where she could sit in it, and when we did she would drink it in with the kind of intense and physical pleasure with which someone who had just come out of a desert would drink a cup of water.

After a little reading and as she began to grow tired, we would detour to the chapel on the way back to her room. As I prepared to leave I would get her a cookie and a glass of milk. The whole routine from arrival to departure lasted about an hour and three quarters. It gave her something to look forward to; it structured her day and made it a little more than simply bearable.

If the routine helped her, it helped me, as I have already suggested, every bit as much. When I arrived I knew more or less what I would be doing; I knew, too, that most often she would respond positively to it and that it would really contribute something to her day. When she was first in chronic care, it sometimes demanded a real effort of will just to go into the building. Her condition then was somewhat unstable, and I for my part had not yet established an adequate routine. Once she was moved, however, visiting became relatively easy. I knew how to deal with the institution and felt at home with most of the members of the staff with whom I came in contact. The pattern of activity that we followed was clearly helpful. Not having to worry any more about other things I could simply be with her and share whatever on that particular day we were able to share.

I have gone into the detail that I have in regard to the things that I did with my mother in order to encourage others to think about what they might do with their chronically ill relatives and friends. Looking back, the pattern I developed seems now to have been self-evident and natural, and yet it required a little imagination and some trial and error before it took its final form. No one helped me in what I was doing. Knowing somehow that such things were important I simply went ahead and did them.

Individuals and families often feel inadequate in a hospital setting. The environment is foreign and somewhat forbidding. It is the kind of place where only professionals seem to be at home. As natural and perhaps as inevitable as such feelings initially are, one must find ways of going beyond them. Trained health care workers have an indispensable role to play, but so do families. In order to fulfill their role they, too, must learn to be at home in the institutional environment. Only when they do will they be able to discover and actually make the contribution of which they are capable.

When I said earlier that the institution and especially social workers have a responsibility to challenge and to help families to become involved, I was thinking above all of the kind of specific activities mentioned here. People in chronic care are by no means all the same. They have different personalities, different backgrounds and educations. The work they did, the interests they developed, the entertainment they enjoyed vary tremendously. Such differences are compounded by their varying states of present health. It is only when the technical and medical knowledge that the institution has is brought into creative relationship with the personal sensitivity and awareness of family and friends that a genuinely helpful program of activities can be developed.

There are two extremes here that one needs to avoid. It might be argued, on the one hand, that it is simply enough to visit and to let things happen in whatever way they might. For some residents and for some visitors, especially for those who are not there very often, this may indeed be true. There can be no questioning the immense value of simply spending time with the chronically ill. Crucial, here, of course, is that one relax and sit down and give them the wholehearted attention they crave and deserve.

Having specific things to do, however, has its own importance. Activities of various kinds can stimulate the mind and the imagination, the senses and the memory of the chronically ill. Sensory deprivation is not an uncommon phenomenon among them. It often results in a confusion between dreams and reality and in an almost paranoid interpretation of what is happening around them. We all need stimulation. For some, television helps; for others it is nothing more than a continuing and confusing blur of image and sound. Doing things with the chronically ill focuses their attention and enables them in some cases, at least, to achieve a better hold on reality.

Having a pattern of activities not only helps the elderly and the ill, it makes visiting a great deal easier. There is nothing worse for families or friends than to come and not to know what to do or say, to feel inadequate if not totally useless. I suspect that some visitors are relieved when they arrive at a room and find the person sleeping. They can at least tell themselves that they fulfilled a certain duty by coming.

The opposite extreme, of course, is to focus so exclusively on activities that one fails to do the one thing that is really essential, that is, to be present to the person and to relate to him or her at whatever level one can. People who are seriously ill and above all those in chronic care often feel a sense of abandonment and of isolation. They tend to try to cope with their situation by withdrawing into themselves and into their dreams and fantasies. This can be a positive thing to the degree that in doing it they are, as it were, regrouping their forces in order better to impose some kind of order and meaning on their new experiences. Carried to an extreme, however, it can reinforce a sense of unreality and of profound loneliness.

A major concern of family and friends should be to draw the person out and to help her once again to experience herself as capable of conversation and of relationship. Such an experience strengthens a person's sense of self and of dignity and worth. As much as the activities that I was able to do with my mother had a value in themselves, they were above all occasions and means for facilitating a deeper and more healing exchange between us.

To stand back and to look at a mother or father in a

chronic care situation can be depressing and paralyzing. It is only as we become involved with them that this begins to change. In the great majority of cases we can, with a little effort, reach them and influence the way they experience themselves and their situation. There are times, however, when this may seem either not to be possible or to be doing so little good as to be hardly worth the effort. It is then that we need to be patient and to trust that at some level something of value is taking place even when we cannot see it. We might learn from the example of the sower in the gospel parable who was generous to extravagance with his seed in the hope that some at least would take root and bear fruit.

Although I had not reflected on it ahead of time, it was impossible for me to become as involved as I did with my mother in her illness without at the same time becoming involved with a good many other people. By coming every day I gradually got to know the other residents on the unit. At noon, especially, many of them used to sit in the corridor. The so-called Golden Rule took on a slightly different twist. It seemed natural to treat them the way that I wanted other people to treat my mother. Or to take another biblical saying, what I did for them I somehow did for her. Their shared pain and disability seemed to create a special bond of solidarity among them.

The more I succeeded in developing relationships with others, the richer my visits became. They, as well as my mother, were able to benefit from my visits. This made what I was doing even more worthwhile and rewarding.

What I did more than anything else with my mother was to build on her strengths. I found what she could still appreciate and enjoy and focused on that. Visitors tended too often to see only what she had lost, what she was no longer capable of doing. When they were unable to go beyond that, they went away saddened and depressed. My experience was a very different one.

Learning to cope with the institution and becoming involved in a deeply personal and positive way with my mother in her new situation went hand in hand. They tended, in fact, to condition one another. Progress in both areas gradually transformed what in the beginning had been for me a depressing and negative experience into what I can only call a time of grace.

4. A Time of Grace

A play I saw during my mother's illness seemed to embody the prejudices if not the fears that many of us have in regard to chronic care. It was about a woman and about her more or less self-destructive relationship to a man she had married when she was young. Although he left her soon after, he continued to torment her throughout her life. By the end of the play she is old, sick, and institutionalized. A great-niece who visits becomes frustrated and angry when she is not recognized and when the old woman persists in talking about what seem to her to be irrelevancies. The woman's one-time husband encounters her by chance in the hospital. Moved by what we are supposed to think is pity, he gives her a gun. The play ends with her suicide.

Sitting in the darkened theater, isolated from the rest of the audience by the intensity of my feelings, I could understand and even empathize with every twist and turn of emotion that was being played out on the stage before me. I, too, had felt anger and frustration; I, too, had been overwhelmed by pity. There were times, especially in the first months, when my mother's suffering seemed so senseless that I could only long for her release.

As much as anger, frustration, and pity are part of most people's experience with chronic care, however, they by no means tell the whole story. As I left the theater that evening I was saddened by the realization that the one-sided presentation I had witnessed was probably the experience of the playwright as well as of some of the audience. During the play's final scene there had been an emotional surge that leapt through the theater suggesting a sudden complicity in fear.

We are an aging population. The more successful we are in dealing with heart disease and cancer, the greater probability there is that more of us will live on into old age. Inevitably chronic care will become far more common. It is crucial that we learn to approach it with other feelings besides fear.

As I reflect on and try to bring together the myriad experiences of my mother's last year, the phrase that persists in coming to mind is "a time of grace." As paradoxical as it sounds, it really describes what in the final analysis the whole experience meant for me. I believe that it also evokes something of what at the deepest level it meant for her.

I speak of the possible positive meaning for my mother of her last months with hesitancy and yet with a certain confidence. If there is something ineffable about all profoundly personal experience, this is even more the case as one confronts death. We talked a great deal, of course, but even more was communicated by silence. The long hours spent together created a bond of understanding and of shared feeling that went beyond anything that we had known before. Here, if anywhere, it is true to say that the heart has its reasons that reason itself cannot plumb.

Mother initially was afraid of dying. Her extraordinary vitality rebelled at the possibility of being extinguished. No matter how profound our faith may be in a life beyond this one, death threatens and destroys the life that we know. As natural as death is in one sense, it remains, in the language of the Bible, the final enemy.

As death became more familiar she was less afraid of it. The challenge then was to live in its presence. What made this more difficult was her reduced state. As long as she was able to make some kind of physical progress, as small as it might have been, she had a sense of life winning out over death. It was not long, however, before obvious limits were reached.

Mother went through the various stages that are often associated with severe illness and death. In the early months she was often depressed. For a long time she found it very difficult to accept what had happened to her. Again and again she asked to be taken home or to church. Several times she said she wanted to go to Ireland for the summer. Many of her fantasies or waking dreams had to do with travel. Slowly, however, she adjusted to what could not be altered and even grew accustomed to being in chronic care. As she did so, subtle but real changes took place in her attitude.

As long as mother had been active, determination and will were among her more prominent characteristics. It had always been easier for her to give than to receive. Intimacy was not something that came easily. As she had grown older, she appeared to me and to others to mellow and to be more at peace with herself and with those around her. What had thus begun continued during her last year. As the weight of her depression lifted she achieved a remarkable level of self-acceptance. Most surprising for me was the fact that she became more at ease with her feelings and more willing to express them. This was something that others noticed as well.

I had always known that my mother was a woman of deep emotions. Within the intimacy of the family their very strength had made them at times somewhat threatening. There was, for example, a sense of intensity about even the way that on occasion she kissed us good night that frightened me as a child. I remember, too, how my father shortly before his death talked about her relation to all three children. She had ways of dealing with them, he said, that had bothered him, but rather than say anything, he had chosen peace.

During her illness mother talked about emotion in general and about her own emotions and how she had tried to live with and express them. It was her mother, she said, who made her afraid of emotion. She had called it, somewhat derogatorily, "sentiment." Dead at the age of fifty before my mother had even married, my grandmother had had a large family and been obliged to struggle to survive when her husband's business collapsed. There were tensions between her and her husband to which my mother referred, but the exact nature of which I did not understand. My mother clearly identified in this area with her own mother.

It was from the same source that she inherited her ambivalence about men. One day during lunch I went out to help one or two of the other women patients and ended up chatting for a moment with some of the nurses. Whether the reference was to the staff or to the residents or to both, mother suggested that really all they wanted was to have a man around. "Not you," I said, and she agreed. I pointed out how ironic it was that in spite of what she seemed to think of men, her children were all males. Not only that but the two who survived were being extremely good to her in her illness. I even reminded her that if my father had still been alive he would have been there every day and would have been very supportive of her. She agreed and confided that in her own life, in fact, men had often been more kind than women.

It was early in her illness and when she was still depressed that one day she said suddenly, "Music is the expression of emotion." I know that we were listening to something at the time and probably talking about it, but I do not really recall anything but the actual phrase and the fact that it erupted almost violently into the conversation. In its suddenness and forcefulness it seemed somehow to have been wrenched from her unconscious. Music, she was saying, was the way that she had dealt with her own emotions. Because they could be expressed in it they were not turned in self-destructively upon her but were given a positive and creative outlet.

On another occasion as we listened to and discussed Chopin we once again broached the theme of emotion. I marveled at his sensitivity and she at his strength. Realizing perhaps for the first time how similar our tastes and feelings were, she said with an enormous sigh, almost a sob: "We are so much alike." It was like a revelation for her. Although in certain respects I had always known how much we had in common, in the course of the year I came to understand it in a new way. Our similarity was probably a factor in the distance that existed between us in the past. If she had inherited a certain diffidence about emotion from her mother, in all likelihood I had inherited the same thing from her. What we shared was not a lack of emotion, but a reticence in expressing it.

The months that mother spent in chronic care were by no means for her a simple holding operation. Life went on. It had entered a new phase, one which like all the other phases before it had its own contours, its own distinctive challenges and opportunities. She continued to grow, to adjust, to cope. She entered into a new level of relationship with me and in analogous ways with other people. She came to know and accept herself in a manner that she never had before. She experienced the truth of her religion in a much less verbal and in a much more personal way.

If in spite of all the drawbacks good things were able to happen to my mother in her final illness, this was even more the case with me. It was, of course, not easy to fulfill the commitment that I had made. I had to juggle my schedule, give up lunches with colleagues and friends, miss a few of my favorite art shows, put up on occasion with professional insensitivity and even, at times, with institutional incompetency. Above all I had to run the gamut of emotions from anger and despair to hope and tenderness. For the first several months it seemed as if I were on an emotional roller coaster. Gradually, however, it leveled off, and although the routine that had been developed continued to be demanding it made my involvement easier and eventually emotionally fulfilling.

For me the last year of my mother's life was in a very special way a time of grace. Although I was aware of this to some degree as it unfolded, it only really became clear how much this was the case as she was dying. To a totally unexpected degree I had come to know and appreciate her. Where before there had been great distance, there was now a strong sense of intimacy and unity.

As with most families, ours too had its emotional complexity. As kind and gentle as my father was, he was no match for my mother when it came to strength of emotion. A kind of feminist before her time she found it difficult to be at home and to channel her energy into small children. Soon after a first pregnancy failed to come to term, she gave birth to my older brother. A little more than five months later she was pregnant with me. When my younger brother was born I was not yet four. The fact that mother almost died at the time and was confined to bed for a year afterward bathed that event and everything surrounding it with an emotion of particular intensity.

Out of this common background each son developed in a slightly different way. Years later when we compared our experiences, we were struck by how varied they were.

Each of us seemed to have had a different mother and above all a different father.

In dealing with emotions and especially with what can be recalled of those of early childhood, it is difficult if not impossible to distinguish between perception and reality, between one's impressions and what in fact might have been the basis for them. Growth in self-knowledge for me has included a growing hesitancy to speak about what others might have felt or intended in their relationships to me. In spite of their onesidedness, however, my perceptions and feelings were a part of my experience and as such have had a considerable impact on the kind of person that I have become. They inevitably influence the way that I feel and think about others and especially about my parents and my brothers.

Some people seem to go through much of their life with little more than a vague awareness of themselves and of their relation to their parents. For such people the emotions that surface when they have to deal with a mother or father in chronic care can be devastating. The situation often calls for a reversal of roles. It evokes things like dependence and independence, acceptance and rejection. For some, it may be the first time that they have had to face a parent's vulnerability and mortality.

I have always considered it one of the great good fortunes of my life that an inability to cope at the age of thirty-one forced me to seek psychological help. I underwent a form of analysis and within six months had brought to the surface some very deep and negative emotions. These tended to focus around my mother. Justified or not I had a sense of having been rejected almost from birth. By the time of my younger brother's arrival, in my mind at least, I had reciprocated by rejecting her in return. Although my life had

been marked by considerable success, it had always been
haunted by a certain emptiness and loneliness. It was something that I felt more and more during my four years as a
graduate student in Europe. There were times, especially
when the pressure of the academic term was over, that I was
overwhelmed by sadness and by tears.

Through the analysis I came to understand how destructive the absence of a positive relationship to my mother
had been for me. Understanding it I began slowly to learn
to compensate for it.

The purpose of these pages is not autobiographical. It is
to say something about chronic care and about how important families are in regard to it. It is because I believe that an
account of my mother's illness and of my involvement in it
can be of help to others that I relate it. To have any understanding at all of our story, however, one needs to know
something about the kind of people that we were and about
our earlier relationship.

I have always been greatly gifted in my friends. In relation with them I gradually learned to accept myself, to receive from others, to be loved. Like my mother, for years I
found it far easier to give than to receive.

In 1974, when I was thirty-six my relationship with my
mother underwent a major development. I can recall dis-
tinctly that at the time I was restless and once again was
wondering whether I should shift from academics to some
kind of counseling work. I went back to speak to the psychologist with whom I had worked five years earlier. Even as
I did so I knew that something was about to happen and
that it was not what was uppermost in my conscious mind
at the time. He asked me why the priesthood was so important and why it continued to feature in all the options that I
was considering.

That night I had a dream and in the dream there was a

series of wooden alphabet blocks. They spelled P I E S T, "priest" without the 'r'. As I woke in the morning it occurred to me immediately that 'r' stood for religion. I had often thought that I was not sufficiently religious to be a priest. As I wondered about the dream that day and about its possible meaning, I focused almost exclusively on my father. To some degree I had become a priest to please and perhaps even to console him. The man he had most admired in his life was the Irish pastor of our parish. In and through that particular priest's eloquence and arrogance, my father had in some measure been able to overcome his sense of belonging to a somewhat disdained minority. It was strange that in all my reflections I failed to relate in any way the dream and what it was saying to my mother. This was all the more odd because the next day was her birthday and I had already committed myself to drive her to my older brother's home for supper. At the time I still found it painful and unsettling just to be in a car with her.

After dinner the following evening I put to my mother what to an outsider would have seemed an innocuous question. I asked her how old I was when my tonsils were taken out. On a conscious level at any rate I simply wanted a piece of information; it would have helped me to fill in what through dreams and psychoanalysis I had already reconstructed of my earliest childhood. The question struck a chord. Mother became excited and started saying that it was neither her fault nor that of my father. It was in fact the doctor who had suggested it, and because he had been the professional they had gone along with him. I did not really grasp what she was trying to say, and then suddenly it was over. "Is that what you wanted?" she asked almost accusingly. "No," I answered, "I really only wondered how old I was when I had my tonsils out."

Somehow in that exchange something happened. Although it sounds arrogant, the only word for it is forgiveness. I forgave her for something the exact nature of which I did not understand, although it clearly had to do with the rejection that I had experienced as a child. For some reason, perhaps simply because she was depressed at having a second child so soon after the first, she had been unable to establish with me that basic attachment that for most mothers seems to come naturally. What she was thinking of was some specific act that might have been interpreted as abandonment and that was related to my being in the hospital for the tonsillectomy. For me the particular event was unimportant. It was at most a type of screen memory around which a whole cluster of emotions gathered.

What happened in me that evening took place not on the level of mind or will but on that of feeling. It was something that was done to me more than something that I myself did. Whatever the precise nature of the emotions and events that had undermined our relationship, the hostility that I had felt for her for so long was gone. I was filled with a sense of freedom.

The next morning I realized that 'r' stood not for religion but for reconciliation. I had been uneasy about my priesthood because of being so much at odds with my mother and therefore with myself. Christianity preaches a message of reconciliation. "God was in Christ reconciling the world to himself," Paul affirmed. To be ordained is to be entrusted with a ministry of reconciliation. The contradiction between that vision and my deepest feelings had been blatant. Now, however, the contradiction was resolved.

Later that day my mother called me, apparently about another question. "Something," she said, "changed between us last night, didn't it?" I agreed that it had. It was a topic about which we never really talked again. Various remarks here and there made it clear how much she understood and how grateful she was that the barrier had been removed.

A friend to whom I spoke at the time predicted that my mother and I would one day be friends. I laughed. The animosity was certainly gone but so, too, was any deep attachment. We were busy people and we tended to go our separate ways. I had the impression that she herself was happy to have me visit only occasionally. Whether because of what had happened, or because of my education, I always felt that she was a little afraid of me. And yet she enjoyed trying out her ideas about church and clergy with me; she knew that I would always say what I thought.

Behind the facade of sophistication and accomplishments of many people a surprising amount of emotional energy continues even into middle age to go into dealing with one's parents. We are, in ways and to an extent that we hardly appreciate, the product of our mother and father. To different degrees their abilities and talents, their genetic structure, their attitudes and values live in us. The mix can sometimes be explosive and destructive, sometimes marvelously integrated and creative. I was always aware of different sides of my own personality, sides that came respectively from father and mother. As one might expect from all that I have said about her, my more active and above all public side reflects my mother. The quieter, more interior, more spiritual and nurturing aspects come more from my father. Perhaps the greatest gift I received from my mother was a share in her great vitality and energy. It forced me again and again as a young person not to be satisfied with success and recognition but to deal with myself. Her vitality in me took the form of a drive for authenticity. Without it I could never have sustained the effort required to resolve our negative relationship. The fact that I did made it possible for me to be there when she needed me. The circle, in my case, had been completed.

Illness and incapacitation are never to be embraced for themselves. One has to fight against them as effectively as one can. A form of piety that suggests anything else is, at the very least, suspect. Nor should sons and daughters become involved with a parent in chronic care because of what it might give them. To attempt such a thing would be a per- version. It would also be counter-productive. I certainly did not consciously do anything during my mother's illness in the hope of getting something from it, and yet in the end I received far more than I gave.

The word "grace" suggests a gift; it presupposes gra- ciousness on the part of a giver and calls forth gratitude from the person who has received it. The last year of my mother's life turned out for me to be an unexpected gift. By becoming involved with her as deeply as I did, I came to know her, to understand her and to love her in ways that I had never thought possible.

Initially it was her need that drew me out. I was unable simply to stand there and watch her suffer or despair or sink into depression. I found things to do, ways to alleviate her discomfort and to appeal to what in her was still capable of responding. In the first months I did most of the giving. It was a time when she could do little more than receive. As the months passed, however, and above all as her condition became more stabilized, she was able to give in return. She gave of herself; she talked about her childhood and parents, about friends and experiences. The more she gave, the more we had in common, the more we shared. Gradually a re- spectful distance was transformed into a close mutuality. The depth and quality of the bond that was being forged became evident at her death and afterward.

The notion of grace is at the heart of Christian experience. Jesus proclaimed the gospel, the good news, of the coming of God's reign or kingdom. What he seemed to mean by this was that God was at hand and that this divine presence implied salvation, reconciliation, and new life. St. Paul translated much of what Jesus said and did into the language of grace. He described the newness of life that was being offered humanity through the death and resurrection of Jesus as a grace. He said that it was being poured into our hearts by the gift of the Holy Spirit. Paul loved the very word "grace"; he used it repeatedly. It underlined for him how freely, how graciously God had dealt with us in Christ. It is not we, he loved to repeat, who are the source of our own salvation. It comes as a gift from God, and as such it is something in which we cannot glory. For St. John, Jesus himself is grace incarnate. In him its fullness dwells. We are related to him as branches to a vine: what comes to us comes through him. In him we see the model and pattern of life that grace is meant to shape and sustain in us.

To have experienced my mother's illness as a time of grace suggests in a Christian context that it involved an experience of divine presence. The Christian experience of God is always in some way related to the person and destiny of Jesus. It is provoked and nourished by the gift of his Spirit.

For some time now religiously sensitive people have spoken of the silence or eclipse of God, even of God's death. I have certainly felt as well as understood the kind of experiences to which such phrases point. The twentieth century, both in its successes and in its failures, has tended to undermine our sense of God. Its success has been largely in the area of science and technology. In the latter, in particular, the emphasis is on ourselves and on how we can manipulate and control nature. The world that we encounter today is rarely free of the imprint of our own hands. Even nature's

most threatening aspects are to some degree the result of
our abuse of it. Nature no longer speaks to us of its creator
with either the clarity or the directness that it once did.

On the negative side, nothing has more marred our
century than its violence. The two world wars and the innumerable smaller ones that succeeded them have destroyed
tens of millions of lives. The holocaust, the systematic
murder of six million Jewish men, women, and children,
reveals the extent of the evil and destructiveness of which
even the most sophisticated nation is capable. Violence dis-
torts in us the image of the creator, while innocent suffering
undermines a sense of his presence and concern.

For many us today the only possible approach to God is
through the human. By entering as deeply as we can into
what is most authentic about our life, we begin to suspect
the spiritual depths that are there. Within us there is a capacity and a longing for what transcends or goes beyond the
realm of daily experience. It is a kind of spiritual energy that
reaches out beyond the self to the infinite. This mysterious
horizon within which we live is what religious people call
God. What is important here is not so much what we do as
the depth at which our activity engages us. Falling in love,
giving birth to a child, taking a courageous moral stand,
having a profound aesthetic experience, reaching out in a
way that costs to someone in need: these and similar experiences reveal the depths of our humanity. They can mediate
an experience of grace.

This was the kind of experience that my mother's illness
became for me. By being as close to her as I was, I somehow
entered into and shared what she was going through. I felt
her frustration and weakness, her depression and confusion.
Most of all I felt the presence of death. It made everything
else that I had to do throughout the year seem relatively
unimportant. To return to the university and to my work

after visiting her and to have to confront the petty concerns and politics that are so much a part of academic and church life was both difficult and depressing. I really felt most of the time that I was living almost as much on the edge of existence as she was. Over that edge there is either nothingness or fullness; my experience was one of fullness. It is to that experience that I am referring in a special way when I say that my mother's last year was for me a time of grace.

For Christians the story of Jesus illuminates and makes explicit what is already implicit in all of life. The God of our heart, the God who stirs our conscience and heals our will is revealed in the human face of Jesus. His life of fidelity and of self-giving love makes visible the invisible mystery of the divine. It offers us at the same time an example or model for what we might be. The Second Vatican Council referred to Jesus as the perfect human. Those who draw near to him, it said, cannot help but become themselves more human.

The way in which most Christians ordinarily try to draw near to Christ is through what they variously call holy communion, the Lord's supper, or the mass. The most widely used term for referring to it today is the eucharist. Under whatever name, the ritual includes two basic components: readings from the Bible and especially from the gospels, and a liturgical reenactment of the words that Jesus said over the bread and the wine at the last supper.

The eucharist became for me more meaningful than ever during my mother's illness. In the acute care hospital, just a few days after the stroke and when she was still very close to death, I celebrated it in a simplified form at her bedside. It was the first of several such celebrations. By recalling and ritually rendering present the suffering and death of Jesus, it bathed her suffering and death in a different light. It gave them a deeper meaning and a heightened dignity. She entered into what we were doing and re-

sponded to the prayers. It meant as much to her as it did
to me.

As we prayed together I remembered another occasion
when I had done the same thing. It had been with my
brother when he too was dying. I had just come back from
Europe to be with him. We talked that day and in the course
of our conversation he was able to resolve certain concerns
that he had. When I volunteered to say mass and asked him
what text from the scriptures he would like to hear, he chose
one that spoke of love and of how when love is present there
is no room for fear. As I read it, tears poured down my face.

During my mother's illness I cried more when I celebrated the eucharist with her than at any other time. Ritual
slows one down and creates a special kind of space and time.
I was more at one with her then than when I was busy doing
things for her. The eucharist brought home that the bond
between us involved divine as well as human dimensions. As
"communion," the whole point of the eucharist is to foster
a bond of unity among those who celebrate it. When we
come together and share in the life and love of Christ, that
sharing is meant to deepen the relationships that exist
among us. Conversely, in drawing closer to one another, we
are able to experience in a more human way what the eucharist is intended to foster. In the eucharist we actually pray
that "we who are nourished by his body and blood may be
filled with his Holy Spirit and become one body, one Spirit
in Christ." These words describe another aspect of the grace
that I experienced in my relationship with my mother during her final illness.

I recently acquired an unusual piece of contemporary
art. A photograph, it juxtaposes the Christ figure from a
well known sixteenth century altar piece with a rather dark
and somber view of the Brooklyn Bridge and of lower Man-
hattan. The wide black border that surrounds the central

images includes the embossed phrase, "Gothic Lament." From an artistic point of view it represents what is called appropriation. From a more explicitly religious and theological perspective it suggests what is meant by living tradition. The church exists to keep alive in changing cultural and social contexts the memory of Jesus. It is a memory that is both consoling and challenging.

In late medieval Europe the suffering and death of Christ were often depicted in gruesome detail. This was a new development in the history of Christian art and seems to have been provoked by the plague. It was almost as if one wanted to say to those who were suffering so horrendously that Jesus had been there before them. No matter how terrible their experience his presence to them in it gave it meaning and dignity. The Christ in "Gothic Lament" was part of a much larger and more complex work that had been painted by Grünewald for a monastery associated with a hospital.

By juxtaposing the Christ of Grünewald with a scene evoking the dark side of modern large city living, the artist invites us to read the story of our suffering against the grid of the suffering of Jesus. This was what mother and I were doing in our celebrations of the eucharist. At some level she understood it as well as I did and was clearly consoled by it.

The eucharist, however, is as challenging as it is consoling. By rendering present the self-giving of Jesus, it challenges us who share in it to give of ourselves. This is what I tried to do with my mother. I gave of my time and imagination, my feelings and energy. Giving all of these I gave something of myself. If, by presenting us with the ideal of Jesus as the man for others, the eucharist challenges us to live in a certain way, it also enables us to do it by the gift that it imparts. The gospel is not primarily a law or even a moral ideal. It is the proclamation and the communication of

God's graciousness, of the gift of the Spirit by which we are to be renewed.

The word eucharist means thanksgiving or gratitude. The Greek word from which it comes includes the word *charis* or grace. Eucharist is a response to a prior gift. We give thanks because we have experienced grace. The grace or gift for which in a special way we give thanks in the eucharist is the gift of Jesus himself and the gift of the life that is made possible through him.

The longer I was involved in my mother's illness, the easier in some ways my role became. This was partly a result of the routine that I had developed. It also reflected the fact that I, like her, was adjusting to her state. As important as these factors were, however, they did not explain for me all that was happening. In Christian language I experienced my efforts as carried and in some way made possible by the presence of the Spirit of God and of Christ in me. It was an experience of grace. In giving I realized how much I was receiving. The only possible response to such an experience is gratitude or eucharist.

What was so real for me also touched others. Different people said how pleased they were to be able to help and how in helping they felt themselves privileged and somehow renewed.

The story of one of my nieces is typical. When my brother died in 1975 she was not yet nine. Although we had spent a good deal of time together over the intervening years, we had never really talked either about him or about his death. When her grandmother had her stroke, she found it difficult to visit her. It made her think about her father and his death and about all that she had missed by not having him in her life. Although I knew that it was a real challenge for her, I asked her to commit herself to go to the hospital once a week. The day I took her to show her what to do, she cried, and later that afternoon for the first time we talked about her father and the kind of person he was. On various occasions during the year when I thanked her for what she was doing, she thanked me in turn for having asked her to do it. At university, she said, students tend to be unrealistic about life. Visiting and helping her grandmother taught her about old age and chronic care and other things that she might never have learned. I am sure that it brought her other and more personal gifts as well. For her, too, it was a time of grace.

The experience of grace is never without its community dimension. I have already said how involvement with my mother inevitably meant involvement with other people. Initially this was other patients—the woman in the same room at the first chronic care facility, those across the hall or next door at the second. In both institutions it took a month or two before I succeeded in getting to know the staff and before they really accepted me. As time went by, however, there slowly but surely developed among us a bond of affection.

In Paul's letter to the Ephesians it is stated that grace overcomes barriers, tears down dividing walls, brings together those who at one time had little in common. Out of the most diverse kinds of people it creates a family in which God's Spirit dwells. This, too, was part of my experience especially in the Catholic institution in which mother died. I hope that the sense of oneness and of affection that developed between me and so many people there will continue in some form.

That this aspect of my involvement was not merely subjective is suggested by the fact that some two months before my mother died I was invited to take part in the hospital rounds. Once a month members of the professional staff are called together for an information and discussion session on some aspect of their work. The various units in the hospital take turns in organizing and conducting the meetings. That month the responsibility fell to my mother's unit. Although the topics in the past had always dealt with medical and therapeutic aspects of aging and chronic care, the unit decided to address the issue of patients' families. They wanted to underline the importance of family involvement, to give some idea of the difficulties families face, and to suggest ways in which they might be helped. They asked me to make the major presentation. I was delighted to do so. The effort to think through what I wanted to say to them began the process that has led to the present book.

The opportunity to speak to the staff and to share with them some of my experiences and convictions was itself a moment of grace. It was an opportunity about which a few months earlier I would never have dreamed. Like life itself, grace has its own rhythm, its own time. We experience it within history, within the ongoing flow of our individual and collective stories. One thing leads to another and that in turn to something quite different again. The key is to be open to the possibilities that encounter us and to respond to them in as creative and positive a way as we can.

The last year of my mother's life was not an easy one. It was above all not easy for her, but it was also not easy for me nor for others who became involved with her during it. When I say that in spite of everything it was a time of grace, I am not denying or trivializing the difficulties. They remained and were considerable, and yet they were not the whole story. Good things happened throughout the year. They happened to my mother and to many of us who shared the year with her. Because much of what happened was so surprising and so unexpected, I experienced it as grace. In and through everything, including what was most negative, there was a healing and unifying presence that a religious person can only call the presence of God.

5. Death and Beyond

Death was something with which mother and everyone involved with her had to deal repeatedly in the course of her illness. The initial stroke had been so massive that it seemed highly unlikely to the medical professionals as well as to the family that she would survive for any extended period. There were several times during the first few weeks when we were convinced that she would not last the night. I can recall, however, saying to the doctors that if natural vitality and sheer determination were factors in a case like hers, then my mother probably had more chance than most.

As she slowly recovered over the summer months, the thought of her death was replaced in the forefront of my consciousness by the challenges involved in learning how to cope with her new situation. My primary concern became that of making whatever life was left to her as comfortable and as meaningful as possible.

As much as she was aware of and tried to respond to what I and others were doing for her, she continued to be preoccupied by death. This came out in various ways. There were, for example, days when she was convinced that she had died and been buried. I remember on one occasion her detailed description of how she had been laid out at the cathedral. Her dreams, especially in the early months, tended to be vivid. They often involved drowning. At certain times she seemed to be more at home with the dead than with the living. Once she identified everyone around her, including me, with friends and relatives from the past, all of whom were dead. Sometimes all I could say was: "You don't look dead to me."

The seizure that she suffered at the end of August reminded us forcefully just how close to death she was. She had manifested so much energy and vitality in cooperating with the therapists that we had become temporarily unrealistic about her true condition. This points up one of the more difficult challenges of the whole year: how were we to keep a balance between, on the one hand, preparing ourselves for her death and, on the other, doing what we could to help her live?

Heightened realization of the nearness of death pressured me to double my efforts to have her moved as rapidly as I could from the first chronic care facility. I did not want her to die where she was. I believed that if I could get her into the other institution and if she were to die there the very next day, I would be satisfied that I had done all that I could for her.

The sense of urgency that I experienced about moving her underlined just how deeply at odds I felt with where she was. In spite of the many good things that had happened there, in spite, too, of a positive relationship with the therapists and with some of the nurses, I did not want her to stay there a day longer than was absolutely necessary.

For all its beneficial aspects, the move brought its own difficulties. Above all she had to learn to adjust all over again. Symptomatic of her general state at the time was the fact that it took months before she became consistently clear about where she was. To someone like myself who was there on a daily basis, it was evident that she was in a state of slow decline all fall. I thought she could die at any time; it hardly seemed possible that she would be alive much beyond Christmas. Members of the staff, however, were more optimistic than I was. They had seen people in even worse condition than my mother who had survived for years.

From January to early April her condition was stable. Clearly she had adapted both to where she was and to her reduced state. The routine that I had developed was also having an effect. It stimulated her and above all gave her something to look forward to every day. Although I am certain that by this time she had accepted death, she seemed to be more involved in life. Death was still mentioned in our conversations, but there was less fear, less anxiety than there had been earlier. Her basic attitude was now one of trust. In the first months when she was most upset, I had encouraged her to use a phrase from the gospel. On the cross Jesus had prayed: "Father, into your hands I commend my spirit." It seemed to me that there could be no more consoling a way to face death than with such an attitude. The phrase was, of course, well known to my mother, being one of the so-called seven last words of Christ. In its Latin form, she had sung it in a number of different settings.

As spring came on I began to wonder if those who had been so generous with their time and who had visited so regularly over the year would be able and willing to continue, and, if they were not, to whom I might then turn for help. I also wondered about my own involvement and about how long I would be able to keep it up on a daily basis.

On Wednesday April 5, I arrived on my mother's floor as usual about 11:15. At first glance, everything seemed normal. Lunch was being distributed; a number of the residents were sitting in the corridor; nurses responded in a friendly way to my greeting. My mother was in her chair just inside the door of her room. I noticed right away a little vomit on her sweater. She had often been sick to her stomach before, but it had almost always passed rapidly. Within a few minutes she was ordinarily settled enough to have a drink or even to eat a meal. This was different. She was obviously upset and not at all well. Suddenly she said that she felt as if she were coming apart inside and were going to die. Realizing that this was neither fantasy nor confusion, I called two of the nurses who were close by. As the three of us watched she suffered some kind of attack. Her head lurched back, she turned deadly white, her eyes bulged, she stopped breathing. All three of us thought that she was dead. After what seemed a very long time but was perhaps only twenty or thirty seconds, she began to breathe again.

Had she died at that moment it would have been an enormous shock. As much as I was reconciled to her death, I was not prepared for it to take place that morning. For me it was another gift that she still had thirty-six hours to live.

Soon after she was put to bed she had a second seizure, very similar to the first. Death was clearly imminent. As nurses did what they could for her, I sat beside her bed and wept. There was a sense of sadness and loss in my tears but also of release. She was on the point of becoming free, free from all the suffering and indignity and dependence of the past year. The tensions with which I had lived for so long were gradually dissolving. I would soon not have to worry about her anymore.

As I wept I listened once again to Gounod's "O Divine Redeemer." It was a piece which we had heard many times and which she had once even asked me to turn off because, as she said, its beauty was so exquisite as to hurt. Played now it bathed both pain and sorrow in an unearthly peace.

One doctor thought that the initial incident might have been a mild heart attack; another identified it as a pulmonary embolism. Whatever the cause, the result was that her heart was further damaged. This induced a pattern of breathing that included shorter or longer periods when she stopped breathing altogether. The longer the interval, the more intense the effort required to begin again. It was as if someone were kick-starting a motor. The violence to the system that was involved was considerable. It was not easy to watch.

Mother's doctor was extremely helpful. He gave us all the information that he had and made sure that we understood the options that were available. The family had agreed from an early date that nothing special was to be done simply to prolong her life. I certainly, for my part, did not want her taken at this stage to an acute care hospital. It was in this hospital and in this room that over the last months she had fought her final battle and had discovered some joy in the midst of her disability. I did not want her to die anywhere else. She had lived a full and rich life and she deserved to be able to die in relative tranquility.

I stayed with her all that afternoon, but that day as every day life went on. I was committed to giving a talk that evening in a series sponsored by a local theological college. It was something that could not be canceled without inconveniencing a number of people. I did what my mother would have done. I fulfilled my obligation. Fortunately, the paper had been prepared well ahead of time.

My niece and my brother took turns being with her until I came back around 9:30. I spent a few more hours with her that evening and then most of Thursday. Although we did not talk a great deal, it was clear that she was quite aware of her condition. She knew that on one of the occasions when she stopped breathing she simply would not start again.

Much of the time that I was there she slept. She was in fact remarkably peaceful. Once she asked me to pray with her. At other times I was able to get a little liquid into her by using a straw as a kind of eye-dropper.

The hospital staff were uniformly helpful and considerate. While respecting our privacy, they were more than willing to do anything we asked.

At the end as throughout her life, music had its part to play. We listened to Bach more than to anything else, and especially to some of his religious cantatas. I remember two in particular. The one for Easter celebrates the mystery of Christ's death and resurrection and with it the larger and more universal drama of death and life. Because of Christ, it sings, death itself has been swallowed up by life. The risen Christ, like the sun, dispels all darkness and with his grace renews our life.

The other cantata was even more moving. Based on the biblical parable of the five wise and five foolish virgins, it evokes an encounter between the individual soul and Christ. "Sleepers wake, the voice is calling. Awake, the bridegroom comes," proclaims the opening chorus, and the tenor echoes it: "He comes, he comes, the bridegroom comes." A wonderful duet by the soprano and the baritone portrays the meeting of bride and bridegroom. The joyous recognition that ensues makes each exclaim: "My beloved is mine and I am yours. Our love can never be severed."

For some, death means annihilation. We are and then we are not. In the words of Macbeth, we "strut and fret our hour upon the stage and then are heard no more." For others, however, it entails both an end and a beginning. It puts a final period to the life that we have known but it also inaugurates another. The nature of this new life is something of which we can have only the faintest intimation. St. Paul cautioned us about taking our attempts to imagine what lies beyond death too literally: "Eye has not seen, nor ear heard, nor the human heart conceived, what God has prepared for those who love him."

Mystics of every age have claimed an intensity of religious experience that for them is a foretaste of eternity. They insist that their experience is real even if radically ineffable. To evoke it they use symbols and images. Their preferred way of talking about it is in terms of human love. Christian mystics, in particular, appeal to and use the language of that surprisingly beautiful biblical love poem known as the Song of Songs.

Fundamental to the Christian attitude to death is the conviction that the abyss into which we fall through it is an abyss of love. Contact with the holy mystery does not annihilate the human spirit but rather lifts it to a new level of personal existence. Life in God gathers up and brings to fulfillment all that in this life was tentative and disparate and not yet integrated. It implies in a heightened form the kind of intense self-awareness and capacity for self-giving that we associate with the ecstasy of true lovers. The all but heavenly beauty of the Bach cantatas brought these and other thoughts into my mind as I sat beside my mother during her last hours.

Human experience is never purely objective. We always bring something of ourselves to it. How much we bring seems to depend upon how personally we enter into it. This is why we experience death so differently and do not simply bring different interpretations to it afterward. My sense of oneness with my mother, reinforced by the music with its deeply religious message, gave my experience of her death a depth and a power that quite literally goes beyond description.

Art in its many forms has a variety of functions and meanings. Important among them for me is that it can express with a unique intensity experiences that I might have but that I cannot formulate as well. Art that does this reinforces our efforts to give order and meaning to experience; it above all sharpens and deepens it and helps to keep it alive in memory.

Over the head of my mother's bed was a calendar with reproductions of Michelangelo's triumphant Sistine Chapel ceiling. The detail chosen for April was that of the creation of Adam. It portrays the outstretched finger of the creator on the point of communicating to humanity the gift of life. As my mother lay there dying, it spoke to me in a very personal way. Faith in life beyond death presupposes faith in the creator God. As Paul argued in relation to the resurrection, the God in whom we believe is the God who gives existence, the God who brings into being what was not. Because he is a God of the living and not of the dead, those who die in him are caught up into his life.

Although science has taught us an enormous amount about the antiquity, the vastness, and the constitution of our world, although it has given us an insight into the complex evolutionary processes by which that world has arrived at its present state, it falls silent before the persistent "why" of the child. Why, finally, does anything exist at all? It is to this kind of question that in its simple and imaginative way the book of Genesis offers an answer. The ultimate why of creation is hidden in the infinite mind of the creator. We believe that he created out of love and not out of necessity. He made creatures in his own image and likeness in order to call them into relationship with him and with one another. Whatever the power and extent of human rebellion against God, whatever the destructiveness of sin in human life, the creator has never abandoned his creation. He remains present to it and in Christ and through the gift of his Spirit leads it forward to its fulfillment. What is true of creation as a whole is true in a special way of each spiritual person within it. Death marks the end of a journey; it implies a final going home.

I stayed with my mother until close to one o'clock that morning. Most of the last hour that I was there I held her hand. There was very little to say. I knew that she was dying and so did she. The important thing was to be with her. When the nurses on the night shift came to move and clean her I decided to go home for a few hours' sleep. I knew that she could die at any moment but I also knew that she could survive for an indefinite period. I told her that I was going and that I would be back in the morning. As I stood up to leave she held on to my hand with a surprisingly strong grip. "Look," a nurse said, "she won't let him go."

A little after two-thirty a nurse called to say that mother had just died. Initially I regretted that I had not stayed, but as time went on, at least in terms of what it would have meant to me, it really did not matter. The bond that had developed between us over the months was such that not even death could break it.

Although I tried, I was unable to go back to sleep that night. I would have liked to have been able to talk with friends, but I did not want to disturb anyone in the middle of the night. As a celibate I have had to learn to confront many things in solitude. Nothing finally is more lonely than dying; my sharing in my mother's death included the loneliness of my first hours of dealing with it.

In the morning I phoned my brother and other members of the family. My cousin, the doctor who had been so supportive throughout the year and who had been so realistic about mother's state, expressed regret. "I'm sorry," she said. "Over the last few months your mother really seemed to be enjoying life again."

I went to the hospital a little later that morning to pick

up the religious and other articles that had been in her room. I wanted to give them to the various people who had helped us so much during the year. Most of the things had already been taken down and packed. The sense of emptiness that I felt was overwhelming. I met and talked with several people on the staff. They were extremely kind and in some cases wept with me. Then and later I realized what a special relationship had grown up among us.

Priests on the whole tend not to want to preach at the funeral of a parent. It is such an emotional time that many are afraid of breaking down. I can certainly appreciate their feelings, and yet very early on in mother's illness I decided that when the time came I would do it myself. Although consciously I intended to do it for her, on some deep level it was also for me. My way of coping with my mother's death as with her illness required activity. By taking charge and doing something I was able to exert a certain control over what was happening. It enabled me to integrate the experience into the overall pattern of my life.

Many priests had known my mother and they could have spoken with great conviction about the more public aspects of her life, about her music, about her work as a volunteer and as a member of various boards. None of them, however, would have been in a position to speak in a really personal way about her last year and about what being in chronic care had meant for her. The danger with me, of course, was that the very intensity of my involvement in her illness might lead me to concentrate so much on it as not to do justice to the rest of her life.

Five years before her stroke mother had arranged and paid for her funeral. She picked out the coffin and even wrote the brief death notice that was to appear in the newspapers. The one question that my brother and I had was whether the coffin should be open or closed. The tradition in our area with people of my mother's generation is for an open coffin. There are arguments of a psychological nature in favor of such a practice. It can bring home to family and friends who were not able to be with her when she died that she is indeed dead. On the other hand the kind of beautifying of the corpse that sometimes takes place can distort in a really unhappy way the memory that one has of the person. We agreed to have the undertakers prepare for an open coffin with the proviso that we would examine what they were able to do and only then make a final decision.

When the funeral director read mother's instructions we were surprised and delighted to discover that she had foreseen and resolved our dilemma. The coffin, she had written, was to be closed except for the family.

When the time came for those who wanted to view the body to do so, I decided against it for myself. I had so many wonderful memories of my mother, including in particular those of the last year and of the last thirty-six hours of her life, that I did not want them distorted by what even the most qualified and best intentioned mortician might have produced. Others, I know, would judge differently; that this was right for me I am absolutely certain.

The one thing that both my brother and I were concerned about for the funeral was that there be good music. We felt that anything less would be an insult to her memory. We need not have worried. People with whom mother had worked in the past came forward and in two days were able to put together a program in which she would have taken real delight.

Many friends said subsequently that the funeral was a genuine celebration of both her life and her death. There were more than five hundred people present including dozens of priests and two bishops. It took place in the parish in which she had lived and worked and prayed for the last

fifty years of her life. Thanking everyone at the end of the
mass, the phrase that spontaneously came to mind was:
"Mother would have been pleased."

A colleague later reminded me that a few months earlier when her father died she had visited my mother and told
her that I would be looking after the funeral. Mother had
responded: "Dan always does a good funeral." I am grateful
that I was able to do one for her as well.

We all mourn in different ways and according to different rhythms. Those who are unable to do so at the actual
time of a death usually do it later. There was for me an
element of mourning in much that I did throughout my
mother's last year. I mourned the diminution of her
strength and vitality, the loss of her independence and
music-making ability. In the last thirty-six hours I mourned
her death.

When those close to us die there is a sense in which we
all die a little with them. The death of one's parents, especially when we ourselves are in middle age, marks a definitive passing of a generation. We now are in the front rank of
our family's continuing journey. Inevitably we become
more conscious of our own death and by that fact of the
preciousness of our children.

If Christian faith proclaims a belief in life beyond
death, it in no sense denies the unique significance that
children can have in reconciling us to our inevitable passing. We live in our children and in their children, as the
Bible would put it, unto the third and the fourth generations.

As a priest and a celibate this is something that I will
never know in regard to children of my own. It is, however,
something that I have experienced in relation to my parents.
I always felt a special bond with my father. Years ago when
my negative feelings toward my mother finally abated, it

was, paradoxically enough, the qualities that I had inherited from him that seemed to come into their own. Feeling more at peace with myself, I felt more at one with what had come to me from him. Something analogous had happened over the past year. Growing closer to my mother, understanding and appreciating her better, I came at the same time, and without even thinking of it, to understand and to appreciate what I had received from her. The end result was that by the time of her death I had the same kind of feeling of unity and reconciliation with her that I always seemed to have had with my father. If both live in God, they also, although in a different way, live in me.

When I went back to the hospital on the morning after my mother's death, tears flowed freely. The same thing happened a number of times over the next day or two, especially when I talked with friends who knew of my involvement over the past year and who in their different ways commented on it. A long and deeply personal conversation with a particularly close friend seemed to have a cathartic effect. From then on I was able to deal with all the demands of the funeral home, the mass, the cemetery and the rest.

Friends were very important for me. As someone without a family of my own, I needed people who knew me and who would have the kindness and patience to listen as I talked about what had happened and about my feelings. It was largely as I did this that my grief ran its course. There were many wonderful things in all these conversations. Perhaps the most touching for me personally was the remark of the father of my godson. Now fourteen, David was the youngest child of very good friends. On a regular basis, almost from the time that he was born, I looked after him and did things with him. Over the years we had developed a very special relationship. His whole family was at the funeral and that evening I had supper with them. His father said how pleased and grateful he was for the role model that I had provided throughout my mother's illness for his son. The way he said this revealed how deeply he meant it. He was surely thinking of the possibility that David one day might be called upon to do the same thing for his mother.

Pressure of courses that were just finishing at the university and then of examinations made me somewhat slow in doing anything about a memorial card. My brother encouraged me to use the photograph that had been taken of mother at the organ to mark her fortieth year as an organist in her home parish. It was the same photo that we had hung in her hospital room and then placed beside the closed coffin at the funeral home. A wonderful picture in itself, it had now an additional meaning because of the important role that it had played throughout her final year.

The next step was to find a text to go with it. As I thought about it, I remembered a poem I had studied thirty years earlier as an undergraduate, John Dryden's "A Song for Saint Cecilia's Day." Cecilia is the traditional patron saint of musicians and has always been associated in a special way with the organ. The poem contained a verse that was almost perfect for my purposes:

> But oh! what art can teach
> What human voice can reach
> The sacred organ's praise?
> Notes inspiring holy love
> Notes that wing their heavenly ways
> To mend the choirs above.

An art consultant put me in touch with a free lance designer who helped transform this material into something very special. A Canadian from mainland China, his Irish American Catholic wife had lost her mother a few months earlier. We understood one another immediately. Together we were able to produce a really beautiful and fitting memorial tribute. Various people remarked how well it captured and continued the note of celebration that had been struck at the funeral.

In itself a small thing, the card became another element in the complex process of responding to my mother's death. It was a way of remembering and of honoring what she had been and done. We used it to thank those who had supported us with their prayers and sympathy at the time of her death. Those who had known and worked with her earlier were grateful to have it as a remembrance of her. I was especially glad to be able to take copies to the nurses and other staff members at the hospital. It seemed important to recognize them as individuals and to thank them personally for what they had done for her and for me. Their work is not easy, and it is, if anything, made more difficult by the fact that so many families simply disappear and are never seen again once their relative dies.

Going back to the hospital not just once but several times has been therapeutic. The emptiness that I experienced on the first visit after mother's death soon disappeared. Two different women have already occupied the room where she had been. I have visited them both and felt quite at home as I did it.

The attachment that over the months I came to feel for a number of the patients will not permit me simply to walk out of their lives without so much as a backward glance. It is truly surprising how much a minute or two spent on a regular basis with chronic care patients can mean. Each person is different, of course, and therefore the relationships that can be developed vary. A woman in her fifties who never spoke and who seemed incapable of any kind of activity or even of much interest was often in the corridor outside my mother's room. I always said hello to her and occasionally offered her cookies or candy. While visiting a number of people two or three weeks after mother's death, I dropped in to see her. She was so deeply touched that she actually said: "Oh my heaven, hello." It was the first time that she had ever said a word to me and indeed the first time that she had said anything to anyone in months. Nothing could more eloquently reflect the emotional power in this kind of setting of even the most simple gesture of concern and friendship.

A bond, too, has been established with some of the staff and in a certain way with the institution itself. I respect what it is trying to do and want to assist it in any way that I can. The fact that people often detach themselves from institutions as soon as they have finished their business with them reinforces an institutional tendency toward the impersonal. We cannot reasonably expect those who run our institutions to deal sensitively with us if we refuse to become involved in any significant way with them.

Writing these pages has been an integral part of the experience of the last year. It has given me an opportunity to reflect on it as a whole and to draw together some of its disparate elements. It was an intense and moving period for me. My mother's illness and death involved me in a way that before it began I would never have thought possible. It was a demanding time but also an enriching and renewing one. If I was able to do a great deal for her, I received in the course of the year even more than I gave.

We all need to make sense of our experience. I saw this continually over the past year with my mother. Some of the apparently most confused things she said were, in the last analysis, the result of attempts to fit the strange sounds and activities and people that surrounded her into what she already knew. In my own way I was doing the same thing.

The idea for a book occurred to me soon after she died. The experience had been so intense and brought me so many insights in regard to chronic care, family involvement, and the possibilities for good even in this kind of situation that I thought I should try to share them with others. Health care professionals encouraged me to do so.

Whatever value the book has for others, the writing of it has been therapeutic for me. It has enabled me to work through again all that happened and in a simple but honest way to try to make sense of it. I realize how deeply my experience was colored by my own life and education. The specifics of my relationship to my mother and of the pattern of activities that I developed are uniquely mine. In spite of that, I believe that my story can be of interest and help to others. As different on so many levels as we are, we all share a common humanity. We all have parents and for many of us one or other of them will spend some time in chronic care. I hope that what I have written will encourage others to become involved with relatives who might be in chronic care. I am convinced that such involvement will be in some way for them, too, an occasion of grace.

6. Concluding Reflections

Experts reaffirm what our experience is already telling us. Ours is an aging population. Medical advances and widespread awareness of health issues mean that a larger percentage of people living today will survive into old age and that a growing number of them will need at some time the assistance that only a chronic care facility can provide.

The challenges created for society by the present demographic situation are enormous. This is most obviously true from an economic point of view, but it is also true in terms of attitudes and values. To build the kind of facilities that we would all want is becoming increasingly expensive. It is in some ways even more difficult to find and keep the nursing and other staff that is required to run them. Chronic care, unfortunately, does not seem to be high on the priority list of either government or elements of the health care profession.

If the notion of quality of life is to be taken seriously in regard to the chronically ill, then the kind and extent of specialized care that will have to be provided is considerable. In order to meet their responsibilities, institutions of this kind are going to have to attract and train an increasing number of volunteers. Above all, families will be obliged to become, much more frequently than they are now, a part of the care-giving team.

As important as professional health care workers and volunteers are, my own experience only really qualifies me to speak of the family. In regard to it, I have a number of convictions. The first is that family involvement is essential.

Everything that I saw and did during my mother's illness convinces me that in many cases the family can make the difference between an overwhelmingly negative experience and one that has some element of meaning and dignity about it.

To speak today in North America of what the family can contribute to social and health care issues is somewhat ironic. The family itself is under very great pressure. Divorce, single parent families, childless couples, families whose members live and work at a great distance from one another: these and similar factors create special difficulties when it comes to possible family support for elderly and ill patients.

Individuals and, where possible, whole families will have to decide in a realistic way what exactly they can and are willing to do. It is my hope that, no matter what their family situation is, people will allow themselves to be touched and challenged in a serious way by the plight of those in chronic care. The philosophy that maintains that life has to go on and that we cannot let our plans and ambitions be even momentarily sidetracked by such a thing as the needs of an elderly parent seems to me to be totally unacceptable. If it were to become the common wisdom in society we would be well on the way to losing our humanity.

The onus to draw families into supportive roles in relation to those in chronic care rests primarily on hospital administrators. It is their responsibility to ensure that their institutions reach out and contact families in a manner that will facilitate their involvement. If this is to happen, each institution will have to formulate and adopt a philosophy that includes in its general understanding of its mandate a positive role for the family. Until this is developed and put into practice, families will almost inevitably be objects of indifference if not of distrust. Their presence will be seen as little more than a possible threat to the routine and good order of the hospital.

The purpose of every health care institution has to be to serve the well-being of its patients. What this entails is obviously somewhat different in a chronic as opposed to an acute care situation. In the former, by definition, the average residency period is much longer. The needs, too, are often more psychological and social than medical. Given such factors, any adequate philosophy of a chronic care facility will necessarily recognize and want to foster the specific contribution that families can make within it.

It is important that such a philosophy be included in the mission statement of the facility and that this in turn be put into the hands of patients' families. Just as institutions need to be clear about their purpose and goals, so those who deal with them require criteria by which both to judge them and to determine their own contribution in relation to them.

The real challenge, of course, is to translate the ideals and values of the mission statement into the flesh and blood of the attitudes and practices of everyone on the staff. Unit administrators have a key role here. They are the ones with whom families have to deal on a day to day basis and to whom in a crisis they naturally turn. My initial and rather unfortunate experience in this regard offers a model example of what should not happen. Trying to cope with a parent in chronic care is already difficult enough without feeling that one has to fight the institution every step of the way. Here as elsewhere, the final responsibility lies clearly with senior administrators. If unit heads are incapable of dealing with families, then the task must be given to someone else. This is an area in which social workers can make a significant contribution.

The process of admission of someone to chronic care should include scheduled meetings with the family. A first such meeting might even take place before the patient actually arrives. An initial introduction of family members to the facility could enable them to help make their relative's experience of being institutionalized a good deal easier than it often is.

Such an occasion might well provide the opportunity to meet the unit administrator and other staff members who will be involved in the ongoing care of the patient. Because it is at this time that the basic attitudes of families toward the institution will largely be determined, it is essential that social workers and others be, and appear to be, open and welcoming to them. Even more significant than the concrete information that has to be provided at this time is the sense that they and their concerns are and will be respected. Perhaps the most important thing that could be accomplished at such a meeting would be to communicate to families that the institution recognizes them as part of the care-giving team, and that it wants to help facilitate their involvement.

Given the mental state in which many families find themselves at such a time, it would be naive to think that everything will be understood, let alone retained from one or two brief meetings. All the pertinent information should be available in written form. Opportunities for family orientation should be provided in group settings and above all at a time when most of those who would like to attend would be able to do so. Once families are brought into contact with other families, there is every chance that they will educate and support one another.

Families are often most at sea in regard to the technically medical aspects of a patient's condition. When it comes to medicine, most of us are woefully uneducated. It

is important, therefore, that a good rapport be established
with the doctor and that he or she be able and willing to
meet with family members and explain to them their relative's condition and the kind of therapy, if any, that is being
developed to deal with it. At an early date, families should
be informed of the kind of options that could be available to
them in the case, for example, of any sudden worsening of
the patient's condition. Failure to face such issues early on
could lead to misunderstanding and bitterness when something happens that demands so immediate a decision that
consultation is impossible.

If the notion of families as part of the care-giving team
is to be taken seriously, then their involvement in the ongoing review of the patient's condition should be a matter of
course. A regular visitor is often more sensitive than the
staff to subtle psychological and physical changes that take
place. Anyone really belonging to the team should both be
able to make a contribution and be kept abreast of the activities and perceptions of other team members.

As important as it is that the institution be open and
welcoming, it is equally important that family members be
willing to do their part. The first thing for them, of course,
is to become convinced of how irreplaceable their role is.
Once this is done, they have to find the energy and the
moral commitment actually to perform it. The effort required to take the first step can be considerable. For some
people the problem is coming to grips with guilt; for others
it is learning to deal with anger and frustration. Whatever
the case, family members need to support and encourage
one another. Almost always one person has to take the initiative, coordinate what others are willing to do, and act as a
spokesperson for them in dealing with the institution. Professional staff can do a great deal by helping families to
discover what, given their particular circumstances and

background, is a reasonable program of activity for them. My own very positive experience with the routine that I developed convinces me that some structuring of one's involvement not only is helpful for the patient but can also make visiting much easier for family and friends. It can also be of real assistance to the staff.

One of the reasons I was able to do as much as I did for my mother was that my schedule was flexible enough to allow me to be there at a time when I could be of most help. I noticed that many of those who visited regularly over the noon hour seemed to be either retired or self-employed. As chronic care becomes more common and as the economic and above all therapeutic significance of families is more widely recognized, governments and employers might well think about what they can do to help family members become involved. With a little imagination and good will, work schedules in many jobs could surely be made a little more flexible. The most important thing here as with most social developments is certainly going to be will. Once there is a social consensus about the importance of something, it becomes relatively easy to discover ways of fostering it. The issue in other words is primarily one of attitudes and values. One might think of efforts in this area as a natural extension of the kind of sensitivity that is now sometimes shown to mothers of young children.

The realization that chronic care often entails a reversal of roles between parents and children suggests that what we have here is more than a simple analogy. Young children can be extremely demanding on parents, especially on mothers. Their state of dependence tends, moreover, to last for several years. It is only right that children should be willing to do what they can for their parents when they are in need. Abandoning elderly and ill parents should be as morally unacceptable as abandoning children. This, of course, does not mean that we can do without our institutions. Quite on the contrary. It implies simply that our responsibility does not end when our parents become institutionalized.

My experience with my mother made me more aware of the role that religious institutions can and should play in regard to chronic care. The biblical tradition puts a high priority on concern for the widow and the orphan, the poor and the weak. The development of health care in western civilization was inspired to a large degree by religious concerns. It is only recently that the growth of government with its increased involvement in all aspects of social life has led to a decline in the presence of the churches in the health care field.

I have the impression that this development has sometimes been interpreted too readily by religious people as an inevitable product of the secularization process or of the modern separation of church and state. Church communities, of course, are not required, nor are they able, to provide all the services that they at one time did. This does not mean, however, that they should withdraw from all institutional involvement in this area. It is interesting that as religious groups, who by definition have a concern for the whole person, have handed over the health-care field to secular professionals, there has developed among the latter a deepening awareness of the importance of a holistic approach not only to medicine but also to other social services. Such people are recognizing more and more that a person cannot be divided into a series of disparate areas or aspects that specialists are then able to treat in isolation. A human being has psychological, social, religious, and physical needs, all of which tend to influence one another.

For many people in our society, religion remains the unifying factor in their self-identity. It grounds their value system and helps them at the deepest level make sense of their experiences. The specific challenges that confront people in chronic care make religion and religious support not less but more important. Chaplains have an important contribution to make here and deserve to be seen as part of the care-giving team. Wherever a church or religious community, however, is willing to become involved in an institutional way in the care of the aged and the ill, it can reinforce considerably what chaplains are able to do. The existence of a facility, the very ethos of which proclaims the religious and human values that are precious to its residents, strengthens their sense of identity and dignity. There is no more concrete a way in which the church could affirm its concern for the whole of human life than by sponsoring and supporting such institutions.

For all its positive values, the danger of a pluralistic society is that everything can be watered down to the point where we all become losers. Its genius, when it works, is to find ways to affirm and celebrate differences without creating prejudice or discrimination. Obviously each religious community is going to have to develop its own distinctive means for bringing together its concerns and contributions with those of the state.

Familial language is very traditional among Christians to describe their ideal of community. We are all called to be brothers and sisters of Christ, children of a common Father. The church itself is often referred to as the family of God.

What is true of family involvement in chronic care in a general way is true in an analogous sense for the spiritual families to which we belong. All religions have a social dimension. This is what Christians mean by church. The average individual experiences his or her religion within the context of a local parish. Entry into chronic care should not mean the end of one's relationship to a particular church community. Nor should the parish think of the person who has been institutionalized as simply moving to another Christian community. Being in chronic care is initially for most people a strange and alienating experience. Ordinarily they are in no condition to begin immediately to develop new community relationships. If they are not to feel isolated and in some sense rejected, their parish will have to continue to keep in contact with them. Clergy can play a part here, but so also can former friends and other parishioners.

The sacrament of the sick as it is practiced in the Catholic tradition should be experienced within a larger context of community care and concern. It is only then that it can have the human as well as religious effect of which it is capable. Every sacrament has what is called an ecclesial or community dimension to it. It is in and through the humanity of our fellow believers that the healing and forgiving grace of Christ is mediated to us. We need to be a great deal more imaginative in developing ways in which people in chronic care can experience this dimension of all the sacraments and especially of the sacrament of the sick.

The fact that family life is so much under attack today makes the role of other and especially of religious groups all the more important. Churches need to be more conscious of their responsibilities in this area and challenge and inspire their members to action.

Chronic care is most immediately of concern to those in it and to those who are most closely related to them and/or who feel a particular responsibility for them. In most cases this means spouses and middle-aged daughters and sons. It would be a shame, however, if younger people and even to some degree children were not to be a part of it. The very presence of the young in such a situation can have a wonderfully therapeutic effect. Certainly those who are in the upper high school years and beyond are mature enough to take their turn in whatever program of support and activity has been developed.

There is another reason why we should encourage the presence of young people in our chronic care institutions. It can have an important educational value. The separating of the old and the ill from ordinary family life has impoverished us all. By visiting and helping grandparents, the young become exposed to aspects of life that they might never otherwise meet. Such experiences can sow the seeds that one day will make it natural for them to support their own parents.

My experience has convinced me that efforts by families to support parents and grandparents in chronic care facilities can be a source of considerable good. Most importantly, it can make a substantial difference in the way that the elderly experience the last years and months of their life. No less significant, however, is what it can do for those of us who reach out to them. It can help us to grow psychologically and spiritually. It can be an occasion to deepen a relationship and perhaps even to establish a whole new one with the person that we are supporting.

Individuals can still make a difference. In regard to parents and others for whom we become involved, that difference can be very great, indeed. Our attitudes and actions, moreover, can also influence the wider community. The more that each and every one of us does, the greater chance there is that our society will become more sensitive to, and caring about, the growing community of the elderly and especially of those in chronic care.

Appendix: The Funeral Homily

It is consoling to be able to mark the death of a relative or friend at a moment when the memory of our solemn annual celebration of the death and resurrection of Jesus is still so alive within us. For believers, Easter is a time of great hope and of affirmation. It proclaims the ultimate triumph of life over death; it affirms both the preciousness of all that is and the fact of God's continuing care for it.

My mother, like every Christian, lived her life within the framework of the life, teaching, and destiny of Jesus. Today's second reading (Rom 6:3–11) recalls how in her baptism she was plunged for the first time into the mystery of his death and resurrection. In the simple ritual of water and words a seed was planted, a seed that she, with the help of the divine Spirit, was to nurture so that it might in her life bear the fruit of goodness and joy, of love and service.

Born in Midland Ontario, Dorothy Hinds came as a young woman to Toronto where already in the 1920s, long before Catholics talked about the women's movement or stressed the role of the laity, she exercised a form of pastoral ministry in St. Paul's parish. She was a kind of social worker as well as an organist and choir director. In the late 1930s and early 1940s marriage and the birth of three sons curtailed much of her activity outside of the home but even then she continued to take piano students.

For well over fifty years she was a generous and active member of this parish. Her most visible involvement was in the liturgy. Playing the organ and singing were her special ways of sharing in the mass. She did it almost daily until her stroke a year ago. When I told an old acquaintance of hers on Friday that she had died, he wondered whether she would be playing at the funeral.

The Catholic Women's League was very close to my mother's heart. She took it and its ideals and projects seriously. She knew that if it was to be effective it had to be alive at the local level, and so, although she became involved in the diocesan and national executives, her first love and abiding commitment were directed to the parish organization.

As her family grew up, mother had more time for outside involvement. The variety of organizations and groups in which she served as a volunteer or as a board member reflect the breadth of both her interests and her concerns. The gradually widening circle of her commitments reflected the changing situation of Catholics in the broader Toronto community. The recognition that was given to her work by the Canadian Council of Christians and Jews as well as by the church was for her a source of pleasure and an occasion for deeply felt gratitude.

The seed that was planted in baptism and nurtured by daily sharing in the eucharist produced in her case much tangible fruit. As long as she was able, she remained active and energetic and generous. This should be recognized and celebrated. As important as it is, however, it is not everything. It in no sense exhausts the meaning and the mystery of her life.

There is a strange and paradoxical saying in the letter to the Hebrews. It affirms that Jesus, although he was a Son, learned obedience through suffering (Heb 5:8). The reference is probably to the agony in the garden although it touches a theme that in some way runs throughout his life. God's ways are not always our ways. The wisdom of the world is not the highest wisdom. Success and public recognition can blind us to the deeper truth of personal authenticity before the holy mystery. Jesus taught us to pray: Thy will be done.

My mother had her share of suffering and failure which, if anything, increased as she grew older. In losing her husband some twenty years ago she lost not only a friend but also a major source of support and strength. The death some years later of her eldest son, Tim, hurt very deeply. Increasing physical disabilities over the last several years, while failing to incapacitate her, made an active life more difficult. Through it all she continued to learn and to grow; she became more accepting, more interior, more at peace with herself and others.

The seed of baptism is a paschal seed. The law of its life and development is the law of death and resurrection. "Unless the grain of wheat falls into the ground and dies, it remains alone; but if it dies it bears much fruit" (Jn 12:24).

In March of 1988 at the beginning of Holy Week, mother began what was to be the last stage of her life. She suffered a massive stroke and almost died. The wisdom of the world would have opted for death rather than incapacity. For many people chronic care is an unfortunate appendage to life, with little intrinsic meaning or value.

My mother's enormous vitality and courage served her once again last summer. Helped by talented and dedicated therapists and supported by her family she was able to come back as far as one could. She never gave up.

At the end of August she suffered a seizure of some kind and began a period of slow decline. As difficult as her condition was during the fall, she gradually became reconciled to it and even achieved a certain inner peace. Over the last three months she was able once again to experience some joy in life. Music was a part of it, as was the loving presence of family and friends. She was grateful for the Catholic environment of the hospital and for its splendid chapel to which she loved to be taken every day. The end came relatively suddenly; she was ready, however, and unafraid. Her last hours were made more prayerful by some of her favorite classical religious music.

Experts tell us that we are becoming an aging population. Chronic care will be part of the life experience of many of us. It is crucial, therefore, that we learn to see it in its normalcy and not as some kind of disaster that comes upon us from without. To do this is by no means easy. As believers, however, we have a special source of insight and strength in our faith. The gracious and forgiving God revealed in the human features of Jesus is present to all of life. No moment, whether at its beginning or its end, escapes his reach. Believing this, we ought to be in the forefront of those who involve themselves creatively and lovingly in the care of the elderly and of the chronically ill.

Our culture, our world, tends to focus on the here and now, on what we can measure and manipulate, package and sell. Our sense for what lies beneath the surface, for what goes beyond the horizons of everyday life, is dulled by our basically noisy and frantic way of living. It is not easy to break out of fixed patterns, but break out we must. The cry of those in need can help us. It appeals to and draws upon what is best in us. It mobilizes our ability to love and to care. As simple as it sounds, it remains true that in giving we receive and that in self-forgetfulness we find ourselves. It is only when we begin to do this that we experience the reality of God. Our own surprising capacities for goodness reveal themselves as his gift.

All appearances to the contrary, the last year of my mother's life was a grace. It was a grace for her; it was a grace, too, for me and for many others who in different ways reached out to her in her need.

May the living Christ, the shepherd and guardian of our souls, lead Dorothy, his servant and friend, to the fullness of eternal life.